"This comprehensive text provides the information you will need to decide which trails to run, how to get there, and what you will encounter on your journey."

—NANCY HOBBS,
Executive Director All American Trail Running Association (AATRA),
Coauthor, *The Ultimate Guide to Trail Running*

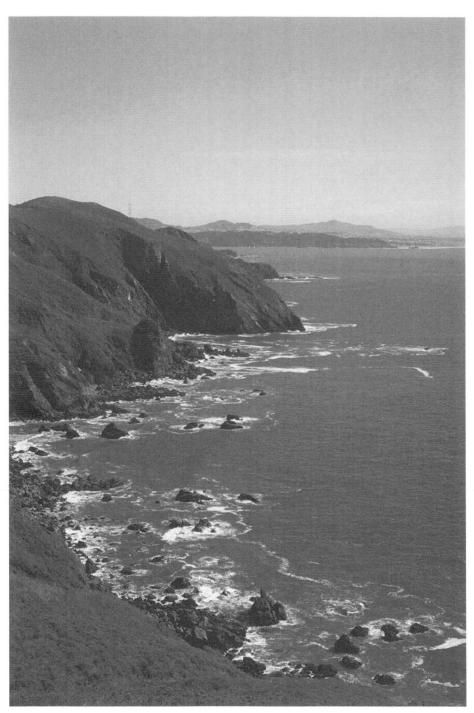

Marin Headlands

50 Runs Around the Bay

TRAIL RUNNER'S
GUIDE
San Francisco Bay Area

Jessica Lage

WILDERNESS PRESS ... *on the trail since 1967*
BERKELEY, CA

Trail Runner's Guide San Francisco Bay Area

1st EDITION 2003
  2nd printing 2007

Front cover photo copyright © 2003 by Marc Muench
Back cover & frontispiece photos copyright © 2003 by Jessica Lage
Interior photos, except where noted, by [Author]
Maps: Jessica Lage and Ben Pease, Pease Press
Cover design: Jaan Hitt
Book design: Courtnay Perry
Book editor: Kris Kaiyala

ISBN 978-089997-309-8

Manufactured in the United States of America
Distributed by Publishers Group West

Published by: **Wilderness Press**
                1345 8th Street
                Berkeley, CA 94710
                (800) 443-7227; FAX (510) 558-1696
                info@wildernesspress.com
                www.wildernesspress.com

Visit our website for a complete listing of our books and for ordering information.

Cover photo: Mt. Tamalpais State Park

SAFETY NOTICE: Although Wilderness Press and the author have made every attempt to ensure that the information in this book is accurate at press time, they are not responsible for any loss, damage, injury, or inconvenience that may occur to anyone while using this book. You are responsible for your own safety and health while in the wilderness. The fact that a trail is described in this book does not mean that it will be safe for you. Be aware that trail conditions can change from day to day. Always check local conditions and know your own limitations.

ACKNOWLEDGMENTS

My family and many friends supported and assisted me throughout the process of this book. I could not have done it without them. Thanks go foremost to Ann Lage and Katie Lage for their ceaseless interest, superlative advice, constant support, frequent companionship, and unrivaled patience. Also to Ray Lage, for his camera, cameos, and support of every kind.

For the many roles they played in the creation of this book, including companionship on the trail, advice, feedback, and encouragement, many thanks to: Leslie Gray, Linda Lipner, Germaine LaBerge, Dan Ruskin, Monica and Eric Axelrod, and Chrissy Meuris (also for her plant expertise and advice of all kinds, including editorial).

Thanks to everyone at Wilderness Press, especially to Mike Jones, publisher, for supporting the idea of a Bay Area trail runner's guide; Jaan Hitt, for her cover design; Matt Heid, for commiseration, understanding, and insights; Jannie Dresser, managing editor, for support, encouragement, and editing expertise; and Courtnay Perry, for her book design and production.

Many thanks also go to editors Kris Kaiyala and Tom Winnett. Tom Ekman, formerly at National Geographic TOPO! provided help with the book's TOPO! maps, and Ben Pease was a pleasure to work with on the locator maps.

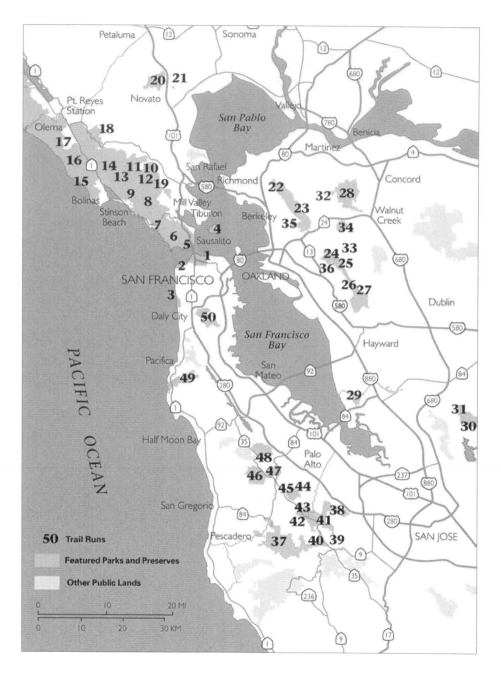

BAY AREA TRAIL RUNS

TABLE OF CONTENTS

HEADS UP!

You are not in Kansas anymore! An important aspect of outdoor adventuring is the presence of potential dangers and risks. Even in the peaceable San Francisco Bay Area, this is true. Ensure your safety whenever you head outdoors and set out on a trail. The fact that a trail is described in this book does not mean that it will be safe for you. Trails vary greatly in difficulty and in the degree of conditioning and agility you need to enjoy them safely. Routes may change and trail conditions may have deteriorated since this book was published.

You can minimize your risks by becoming knowledgeable. Know where you are going and what variables you might encounter. Be prepared and alert. Although we don't have bears in the Bay Area anymore, and tigers are not native to North America, we do have an occasional mountain lion sighting. We also have poisonous plants, dangerous road crossings, and unfriendly or threatening individuals. There's no way this book can give you a full treatise on outdoor safety, but good books are available and there are classes that cover trail safety, survival techniques, and first-aid.

Know your surroundings and, more importantly, know your own limitations. Anticipate adverse conditions, like the late afternoon downpour that has been predicted even if it seems to be a perfectly sunny day. Tell someone where you are going and let them know when you return. Be prepared to deal with unexpected problems by selecting a different and safer route or by asking a partner to share the adventure with you. Millions of people enjoy safe outdoor adventures every day. As a trail runner, you assume all the risks associated with your chosen activity. Heads up, have fun, and let us know if there are changes you encounter so that we can keep this book as up-to-date as possible.

PREFACE

Many runners speak of running as an addiction: a physical need to work their body, to engage their muscles, lungs, and heart. They equate running with a sense of being "alive." Trail running engages more than just this interaction with your body—it is an encounter with the natural world; you are at once immersed in your environment and fully present in your body.

I yearn for the Bay Area's smells, textures, and views that I experience on my runs: to awake to the Hunter's Moon hanging low in the sky, reflecting off thick white fog over the bay; to brush through dew-damp grasses on a coastal ridgetop; to meet a grey fox on a narrow trail; to drink in the dense, piney fragrance on a forest of Douglas-firs. Exhilarating encounters with the natural world, coupled with the deep satisfaction of physical exertion, are what trail running is all about. Through trail running, you will come to know the Bay Area and yourself in a unique and rewarding way.

Trail Runner's Guide San Francisco Bay Area brings this sport to your backyard, whether you're a local resident or here for a visit. You'll find 50 featured Bay Area trail runs in this book, plus at least as many suggestions for other routes. Narrowing the selection to 50 was not easy. In choosing these runs, my priorities were to include routes that highlight the Bay Area's diverse landscapes and also to offer a range of length, difficulty, and location, so as to accommodate experienced and beginning runners, and everyone in between. The book also includes basic trail running tips as well as safety and equipment suggestions.

This book is for every class of trail runner: those who run for the pure joy of running; those who run to feel the wind on their face, to smell the earth after a rain, to watch the fog roll across the bay; and those who need the enticement of a scenic adventure to put on their running shoes and get out the door. There can't be a better incentive than the vast variety of natural beauty that the routes in this book encompass.

I think of this book as a jumping-off point—an overview of some of the best trails in the area. I hope you will use it to familiarize yourself with the geography, natural features, plants, parks, and open spaces of the Bay Area. Use it to find a trail convenient to your home or work and that can be incorporated into your everyday routine. Use it to experience the thrill of finding a new run and to discover new surprises on familiar routes. If you're new to the Bay Area or a visitor here, use it to discover the world-class beauty of this unique place.

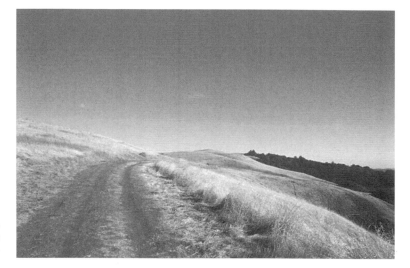

Ridge Trail,
Russian Ridge
OSP (Run 42)

INTRODUCTION

A trail run is at once an athletic and a sensory experience: you are vigilant of your body as well as keenly aware of the natural environment. Your muscles contract and release, your heart pumps, your lungs burn on a steep climb and expand again on a downhill. You are attuned to everything around you—a rock or log in your path, an overhanging branch, overzealous poison oak. Your body reacts quickly as your mind registers the trail's features—steep, level, rocky, smooth, narrow, muddy, slippery, obstructed. Smells, views, and terrain compose your run: You absorb the pattern of rocks in the trail or the low wildflowers lining its edges, and though you may not notice every trailside feature, you incorporate your surroundings into your awareness as you run.

Runners seek out trails for various reasons. Many trail runners choose dirt and rocks over pavement and sidewalk because they thrive on this intimate connection to the natural world. They enjoy the challenge that nature presents: No route is ever exactly the same twice—erosion alters the grade; rains turn a smooth trail into a muddy mess; winds blow down tree branches; seasons bring new smells and new colors. Changes in weather can turn a sweltering, dusty run into a windy, fog-enshrouded adventure in a matter of minutes. Because natural forces so directly impact a trail run, trail runners become acutely aware of their environment—of the cycle of the seasons, weather patterns, and topography.

Some runners seek out trails because their surfaces are easier on knees, feet, and other joints than pavement is. When you run, your body hits the ground with five times more impact than when you walk. Softer and more pliable dirt surfaces do less damage to your joints than concrete and asphalt, which are less yielding and bear greater potential for injury. In addition, because trail gradients and surfaces vary frequently, running on trails engages a range of muscle groups and helps prevent repetitive stress injuries.

Trail runners usually find that time is a more meaningful measurement than mileage. Terrain and conditions influence pace much more than on a road run. A good trail run is determined more by what you encounter or experience—a spectacular sunrise, a breathtaking coastal view, a lung-bursting climb, or a new path—than by beating a personal best.

TRAIL RUNNING IN THE SAN FRANCISCO BAY AREA

The San Francisco Bay Area is a trail-running hub. An active population, a mild climate (70-degree F days in February are common), and an extensive network of trails draw runners outdoors year-round. You can watch wisps of summer fog roll across the bay and cool the afternoon sun. You can enjoy the thick smells of the hard-packed, dusty trails of fall, surrounded by seas of dry brown grasses and spent sticky monkeyflowers. You can brave mud in winter and smell the trails after a spring rain.

You don't have to drive far in the Bay Area to feel like you've been transplanted from urban frenzy to serene natural beauty. Thousands of trails traverse the open spaces that have been carefully set aside throughout the Bay Area's densely populated cities. Regional trails link individual parks and preserves.

The diverse environments within the Bay Area mean that you can enjoy dramatically different views in a matter of minutes on a trail run. In a couple of hours or less, you can encounter unique terrain and pass through a variety of natural communities. In Point Reyes, for example, you can go from Mt. Wittenberg (the seashore's highest peak), through a thick Douglas-fir forest to the coast, and return via a alder-lined streamside trail to an open meadow dotted with oak trees. On Mt. Tamalpais, you might cross an exposed chaparral-covered hillside, enter a shady redwood forest, and loop back on grassy slopes above the coast.

BAY AREA NATURE

The 900-square-mile body of water known as the San Francisco Bay is the defining feature of this geographical region; it includes northern and eastern extensions (San Pablo and Suisun bays respectively). The bay receives freshwater from the Sacramento and San Joaquin rivers that mixes with salty Pacific Ocean water to form the largest estuary on the West Coast.

The Golden Gate, the bay's opening to the Pacific, creates a break in the Coast Ranges—the mountains that rise abruptly from the Pacific. In California, the Coast Ranges run from the Oregon border to the Transverse Ranges (near Santa Barbara); in the Bay Area, the range is a double line of mountains between which lies the bay. These mountains play a major role in the Bay Area's moderate climate. From 2,000 to 4,000 feet high, they act as a barrier to hot and cold air masses and protect this coastal region from Central Valley

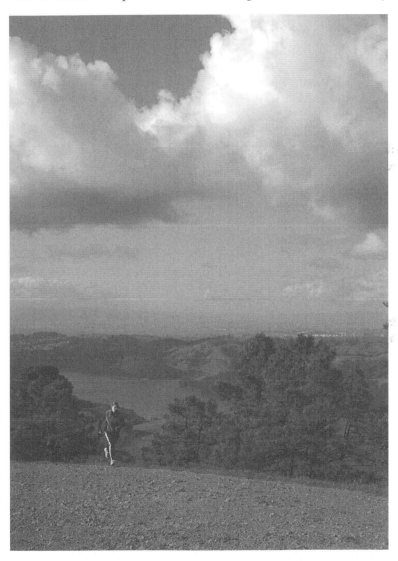

Runner on Sea View Trail, Tilden Park, with San Pablo Reservoir in the background (Run 23)

heat in summer and continental cold air in winter. The relatively cool, dry summers and mild, wet winters of the Bay Area's Mediterranean climate are what makes outdoor recreation enjoyable year-round.

Seasons While it's true that Mediterranean climates lack the dramatic seasonal changes that many parts of the country see, even the Bay Area experiences a distinct seasonal cycle in its own subdued way. You will become keenly aware of seasonal changes as you discover the Bay Area's natural world.

Winter: Early winter—from late December to the start of January—often brings a spell of mild weather, during which temperatures reach into the seventies and often surprise even Bay Area natives. These welcome days can be the best of the entire year—warm and fogless on the coast and not excessively hot inland.

When winter rains come (if not impeded by drought), the rolling hills turn a luscious, vibrant green. Windy storms threaten new blossoms that had already signaled spring. Dark, swollen clouds hang low, and white wisps stretch across the sky; when the rain breaks, brilliant blue skies grace crisp, clean days. The rains often saturate the earth, and trails on the East Bay's clay soil become unbearably muddy.

Delicate pink and white manzanita flowers begin to appear on the low shrubs, and the small tassels of currant flowers cast a pungent fragrance. Wildflowers, especially those on south-facing slopes, begin their spring show. Milkmaids are among the first to appear, with buttercups, sun cups, blue dicks, and blue-eyed grass soon after. Sweet-smelling ceanothus flowers burst into white and blue-purple blooms.

In early March, a few days of unseasonably warm temperatures invariably settle over the Bay Area, raising hopes of winter's end, but often more rain is in store as winter has its last blast.

Spring: Although Bay Area winters often flaunt spring-like weather, spring formally arrives at the end of March when the days begin to lengthen noticeably. New growth bursts out of every nook and cranny of the earth: oak trees put on a subtle but incredible show, with lengthy tassels that dangle from rosy new leaves; lupine, buttercups, poppies, Indian paintbrush, larkspur, and iris coat the hillsides in sensational colors; and vibrant green growth shoots from the tips of

Douglas-firs. The weather is unpredictable, but often breezy and cool, and billowing clouds blow across blue skies.

As spring flows into summer, the hills begin the gradual shift from green to golden. Buckeye trees are in full bloom, and cow parsnip, mugwort, and poison hemlock encroach on the edges of trails. Dry grasses and thistle grow several feet tall and unruly; orange sticky monkeyflowers and Indian paintbrush are out in full force.

Summer: Summer creeps up on the Bay Area, signaled by thick morning fogs; the fog comes in daily and weekly patterns, rolling in from the coast and spreading over the bay and coastal areas. Most days, the sun's warmth burns off the greyness by midday. (Fog is an important element of the Bay Area climate: some areas near the coast and in the hills, where fog often hovers low and dense, receive up to 10 inches of precipitation per year in the form of fog drip.) By June, hillsides are almost entirely brown, yet if you look closely, you will see green among the dry grasses; these are still not the golden hills of October. Orange-yellow sticky monkeyflowers are among the few wildflowers that remain along the trails by summer. Clumps of small red berries abruptly replace the bushy white flowers of the red elderberry, and blue elderberry bushes also begin to bear fruit.

Fall: Fall officially begins in late September, when the Bay Area typically experiences its hottest weather. Indian summer displaces the fog belt, rejuvenating us after the often-dreary, grey August days. The

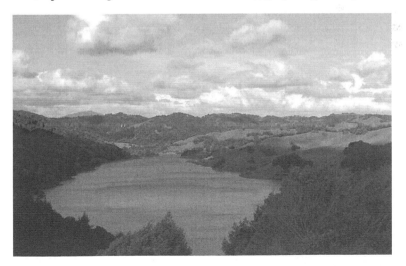

Briones Reservoir on a blustery spring day (Run 32)

cold upwelling in the Pacific subsides, and warmer water dissipates the fog, so the coast is clear and warm. A golden light slants across dry hillsides and through brittle leaves, and poison oak displays the first fall color. A welcome crispness hangs in the early morning air. Trees lose their leaves and fruits appear on bushes: white snowberries hang from bare branches; glossy red honeysuckle berries dangle at the tips of the crawling vines; and toyon berries, currants, and coffee-berries appear. Coyote bush goes to seed, sending fluffy white tufts drifting through the air. Warm weather often continues into November, but the days shorten and winter is palpable.

Climate

As a trail runner, you learn that landforms and weather are inter-twined, and that geography and climate directly influence our expe-rience in the natural world. They are the factors we consider when choosing a trail: the steepness of the grade; whether or not winter rains muddy the trail; the best location for each time of year; whether the route is hot or cold, foggy or windy, shaded or exposed; and the type of vegetation.

This region's diverse topography produces a range of microcli-mates within this a relatively small area. When fog smothers the coast and hangs low over ridges, inland valleys may be bathed in sun; when Marin County temperatures call for shorts and sleeveless shirts, you may find yourself bundled in warm clothing in Berkeley. The Bay Area's microclimates not only influence the way we live, but more dramatically, they affect the plant world around us.

Bay Area Plant Communities

More than 2,000 species of plants live in distinct plant communities in the Bay Area. You'll often pass through many communities on a single run.

Coastal Scrub

On sea bluffs, where wind and fog shape plants into low and tufted sculptures, coastal scrub plants predominate. You'll find coyote bush, coffeeberry, California sagebrush, blossoming lupine, sticky mon-keyflower, sprawling morning glory, ferns, and the ubiquitous poison oak on sandy bluffs in the Marin Headlands and Point Reyes, and on San Francisco's coast (Runs 1, 2, 5–7, 15, and 16).

Coastal Grassland

Coastal prairie or grassland plants thrive just inland from the imme-diate bluffs, where the influences of wind, fog, and salt are not as strong. Willowy grasses, native or introduced, drape the rolling hills,

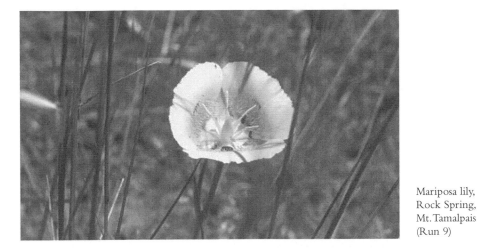

Mariposa lily,
Rock Spring,
Mt. Tamalpais
(Run 9)

often scattered under stands of redwoods or Douglas-firs. Wild-flowers adapted to frequent fog sprout perenially among the grasses: blue-eyed grass, blue dicks, mariposa lilies, and Douglas iris are among the species you'll see on the hills of Bolinas and Russian ridges in spring (Runs 14 and 42).

Closed-cone Forest

In foggy coastal areas, closed-cone pine and cypress forests live on nutrient-poor soils. Bishop and Monterey pines and Sargent and Monterey cypresses are among the trees that grow here. Called "closed-cone" because their cones do not open at maturity, these trees instead require fire or a particularly hot day to open the cones and disperse the seeds. You can observe first-hand the effects of fire on the bishop pines on Inverness Ridge in Point Reyes and their vigorous recovery after the 1995 Mt. Vision Fire (Bear Valley Loop, Run 17).

Redwood Forest

Although redwood trees once covered Bay Area hillsides, today only pockets of mostly second and third growth forests remain. Red-woods grow in moist, foggy environments, anywhere from 1 to 10 miles inland from the coast, removed from salt spray and strong winds. The thick layer of needles, branches, and plant debris that collects under redwoods, combined with the shade from the giant trees, creates an environment where few plant species can survive. Thimbleberry and huckleberry bushes, as well as sword fern, red-wood sorrel, and salal, are some that can grow in these forests. Muir Woods (Mountain Home Loop, Run 8) and Redwood Regional

Park (Runs 24 and 25) are two good places to experience Bay Area redwoods.

Mixed Evergreen Forest

In coastal California, mixed evergreen or hardwood forests often stretch between moist redwood forests and drier foothill woodlands. Live oak, tanbark oak, madrone, chinquapin, bay laurel, and Douglas-fir thrive in these intermediate zones, where the climate is neither excessively hot nor too damp. Buckeye and black oak are two deciduous trees that grow among the more prominent evergreens. A medley of salal, barberry, huckleberry, manzanita, poison oak, and hazelnut grow beneath the trees, depending on the moisture content of the soil.

Riparian Woodland

In canyon bottoms and riverbeds, deciduous trees join mixed evergreen forests. Big-leaf maple, willow, alder, birch, and cottonwood trees flourish in riparian forests. Their golden leaves coat the ground in fall and winter; in summer, their full, leafy canopies create dense shade. Alameda Creek in Sunol Regional Wilderness (Runs 30 and 31) is a rich example of a riparian woodland.

Oak Woodland

Removed from foggy coastal influences, oak woodlands cover the interior rolling hills of California. Hot summers and low winter precipitation encourage a variety of deciduous and evergreen oaks—valley oak, blue oak, black oak, canyon oak, interior live oak, and coast live oak—as well as buckeye and grey pine. Oak woodlands predominate at Mt. Burdell Open Space Preserve (Mt. Burdell, Run 20) and Sunol Regional Wilderness (Runs 30 and 31).

Chaparral

The evergreen shrubs of the chaparral community cover hot, rocky, south-facing slopes throughout the Bay Area with dense, prickly growth. Manzanita, toyon, chamise, shrub oak, ceanothus, coffeeberry, and other chaparral plants have adaptive features that allow them to grow and flourish with little or no summer water, in coarse, dry, and eroding soil. Despite this relatively harsh environment, chaparral communities come alive with color and fragrance: blue, purple, and white ceanothus blossoms scent the air; bright pink wild currant flowers dangle from branches; vivid golden flowers decorate bush poppies; and red toyon berries splash color across chaparral slopes in fall and winter. These evergreen bushes take advantage of winter and

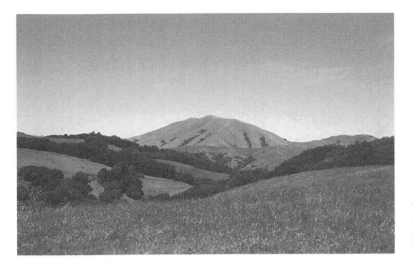

View of Black Mountain from the Bolinas Ridge Trail (Run 14)

spring rains to sprout new growth yet remain dormant in summer, when water is least available.

PLANTS AND ANIMALS TO AVOID

While trail running you're exposed to the best and the worst of the Bay Area's natural world. Here are a few things to be on the lookout for while you're on the trail.

Poison oak is ubiquitous in the Bay Area. You will find this tenacious plant in most every habitat—forests, riparian areas, open chaparral, and coastal bluffs. Know what to look for. Poison oak's appearance can vary deceptively: the shiny, lobed leaves may be very large or very small; they most often grow in clusters of three, although some variations grow in fives. **Poison Oak**

An oily residue coats the leaves and branches of poison oak. Contact with it can result in a blistering, itchy rash. Some people are fortunate enough not to be susceptible to this plant's toxin; others, however, may develop a rash in mere hours or in a week or two. The oily residue is hard to wash off and can be transferred to skin from clothing, fur, and other materials (dogs are notorious carriers). You can contract the oil at any time of year from the shiny green leaves in summer, the brilliant red fall foliage, or the dry, spare sticks in winter. All are potent.

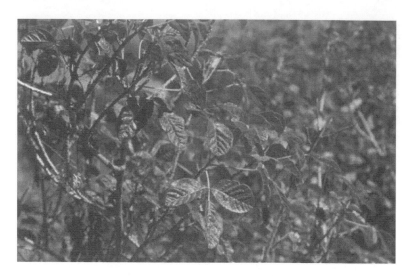

Poison oak

If you come into contact with poison oak, the best antidote is to wash the contaminated area thoroughly with soap. People who are especially sensitive may want to try a soap that is specifically formulated to combat the plant's oil, such as Tecnu Oak-n-Ivy® Cleanser or Ivy Block®. Be sure to wash your clothes and shoes too.

You will encounter poison oak on most of the runs in this book, but don't be discouraged! If you exercise caution, you can avoid touching it. Narrow singletrack trails clearly create the greatest vulnerability. On wide fire roads, watch for overhanging branches.

Ticks   After poison oak, ticks are probably the most common hazard you'll encounter on Bay Area trails. Prime tick season is late spring and early summer. These tiny teardrop-shaped pests (about an eighth of an inch long) live on grasses and shrubs. When you brush against trailside plants, they hitch onto your clothing and make their way to an open patch of skin.

Some ticks transmit Lyme disease, although only 1 to 2 percent of ticks in California are infected with the disease. Try to avoid narrow trails overgrown with brush or grasses during tick season. You can use an insect repellent that is labeled as effective against ticks. Check yourself for ticks after a run, especially warm, moist places on your body.

If you are bitten by a tick, use tweezers to pull out the tick, taking care to remove any mouthparts. If the mouth or head breaks off and remains under your skin, contact your physician. Do not touch the tick, since the "juice" can also transmit the disease. Wash the bite area and your hands with warm water and soap and apply an antiseptic.

Rattlesnakes

Only one native venomous rattlesnake lives in the Bay Area, the Northern Pacific rattlesnake. Gopher and bull snakes are often confused for rattlesnakes because they have similar markings, but a rattlesnake's distinctive thin neck and arrow-shaped head—and, of course, the rattles on the tail (although a young rattlesnake may have a rounded tail)—distinguish it.

The Northern Pacific rattlesnake is not aggressive and strikes in defense or to get food. Your footsteps warn the snake of your presence, and it moves away if it can. Take care to prevent a snakebite by staying on the trail and avoiding tall grass and heavy underbrush. (Also watch for the occasional rattlesnake sunning in the middle of the trail.) Remember that baby rattlesnakes are also poisonous.

If you are bitten, stay calm. Do not walk or run unless you are alone, in which case walk slowly to seek help. Do NOT pack the bite in ice or make an incision in the bite to suck the venom out or apply a tourniquet. Call 911 for treatment as soon as possible. Very few rattlesnake bites are fatal.

Mountain Lions

The Bay Area is mountain-lion habitat. Lions, or cougars, as they are also called, are important links in the natural food chain, keeping the deer and rabbit populations in check. They are elusive, solitary, and usually nocturnal animals. A typical mountain lion may range between 20 and 100 square miles. Human development has significantly altered their habitat and impeded natural corridors; as more people use hiking and running trails along urban fringes and in open spaces, reported sightings are on the rise. Nevertheless, it is unlikely that you will ever encounter a mountain lion, and an attack is even less likely.

Although highly unlikely, if you meet a mountain lion on the trail, here are a few basic rules to avoid an attack:

- Do not run—running away stimulates the cat's predatory instincts.
- Do not turn your back—make eye contact and back away slowly from the animal.
- Do not bend down (you'll look like a four-legged prey).
- Pick up pets or small children immediately (without bending down).
- Stand upright and make yourself look larger by raising your arms above your head or opening your jacket, if you are wearing one.
- Throw stones, branches, or whatever you can reach without crouching or turning your back.
- If approached, wave your arms and speak firmly or shout.
- If attacked, fight back aggressively; since a mountain lion usually tries to bite the head or neck, try to remain standing and face the attacking animal.

TRAIL RUNNING BASICS

Running on a trail presents different challenges than running on a paved road or around a track and requires more concentration. Avoiding natural obstacles like roots, rocks, and overhanging branches requires agility and careful footing. The constantly varying terrain on trails engages different muscles with each step. Although the benefits of trail running greatly outweigh the hazards, there are a few things that everyone, especially beginners, should know.

A twisted ankle is probably the most common trail running injury.

If you are new to trail running, increase your mileage and route difficulty slowly. Look for the shorter routes in this book and those with an easy rating, and read the **Trail Notes** to find out what the trail is like. Begin on wide trails with relatively smooth surfaces. Gradually move to more rugged terrain and more challenging routes. Give your muscles time to strengthen and become accustomed to new demands by slowly increasing mileage and difficulty. Rough terrain and sharp turns tax your body, particularly your ankle tendons.

Running both up and down hills is easier when you remember a few basic tricks: On uphills, keep your body erect—resist the urge to lean forward. Although you may have to walk up long, steep hills, it's best to try to maintain your momentum by taking small steps and continuing at a run. On downhills, keep your body relaxed and stay light on your feet. Shortening your stride and bending your knees can help lessen the impact on your knees by employing your quadricep muscles. Some runners prefer to lengthen the stride and let the body flow freely.

Get used to constantly scanning the trail ahead. Look for roots, rocks, muddy spots, and holes and pick up your feet to avoid them! Also watch for overhanging branches and other surprises along your route.

Shuffling along on a trail is a sure way to fall.

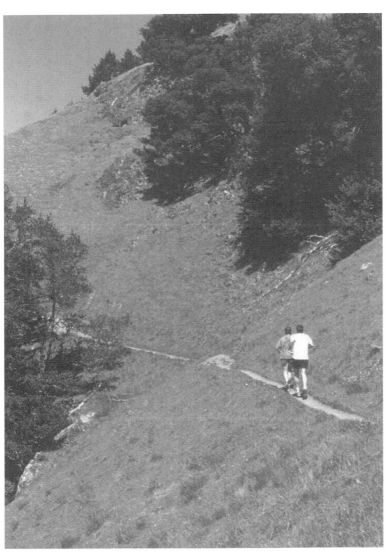

Runners on Coastal Trail, Mt. Tamalpais (Run 9)

Beginning trail runners are not the only ones who seek out smooth, wide trails. Softer surfaces and natural beauty, rather than challenging, rugged terrain, are what draw many people to trail running. If that's true for you, choose your routes accordingly. Many routes in this book feature smooth trails with few obstacles, and you'll usually find options for less-encumbered trails in the **Alternate Route** suggestions. Check the **Trail Notes** section to find out what types of trail the route includes—singletrack or fire trail—and what the terrain is like. The brief summary at the beginning of each route often includes this information as well.

Fire trails and service roads are unpaved, wide, and usually smooth and free of rocky obstacles (with the notable exceptions of Eldridge Grade on Mt. Tamalpais and the Big Springs Trail in Tilden Park). Singletrack trails are narrower than fire roads—just wide enough for one person—but they can vary in width and terrain. Again, check the **Trail Notes** for details. Many runners prefer the interest and challenge of singletracks, even though they often come with added obstacles.

TRAIL RUNNING EQUIPMENT

Much of the appeal of trail running lies in its simplicity: the only essential equipment is a good pair of running shoes. However, a water-bottle or a hydration pack, a pair of sunglasses, a windbreaker, a hat, and gloves may increase your comfort and enjoyment while running.

Running Shoes In the few years since trail running has soared into the fitness spotlight, manufacturers have designed and put on the market about 40 different models of shoes made specifically for the sport. More than a dozen companies, from traditional running-shoe manufacturers like adidas and Nike to companies conventionally associated with hiking, such as Vasque, Merrell, Teva, and The North Face, have added trail-running shoes to their product lines.

Trail running shoes generally afford more foot protection, support, and traction than road running shoes. A multi-layer toebox or an extended sole shields your toes from impact with rocks, roots, and other obstacles. A stiffer midsole provides more stability, and aggressive tread provides better traction on slippery or gravelly slopes; tread is also designed to flake off the chunks of mud that often get caught in road running shoes. Some trail running shoes have a Gore-Tex lining to keep your feet dry on rainy days and when crossing flowing creekbeds. High ankle collars in many trail running shoes work to keep out dirt and scree.

Unfortunately, these additional features usually make trail running shoes bulkier than road running shoes. Also, they are not as cushioned as their road counterparts, and although a softer running surface may compensate for the reduced padding, this is one of the main complaints about trail shoes. If this is true for you, your knees will let you know.

Weigh the advantages and disadvantages of trail and road running shoes, taking into consideration the terrain you usually run on, the distances you run, the number of miles you want to get out of the shoes, and the price you can afford. Although trail running shoes aren't required in the Bay Area, since most trails here don't entail difficult water crossings and icy surfaces, you may prefer the extra protection trail running shoes provide. Consider investing in two or more pairs of shoes—trail running shoes for rockier trails and road running shoes for fire trails and smooth dirt paths.

The most important thing is to find a running shoe that fits you well and is comfortable. Experiment with different shoes for the fit and features that are right for you. Shoes that are worn out, don't fit well, or are not the proper design for your body can cause injuries. It is also important to take proper care of your feet in order to avoid blisters, corns, and bunions.

Your feet are key components of your body's mechanics and receive the brunt of your weight.

Clothing

Trail running doesn't require a lot of special gear, but a few items will make you more comfortable. Remember that the weather in the Bay Area is variable; you may start out in a chilling fog and finish in hot sun—or vice versa. Moisture-wicking fabrics like polypropylene and polyester fleece keep you warm in wet weather or when sweaty skin meets cool fog. Cotton, on the other hand, absorbs moisture and can make you colder or cause chafing. A lightweight windbreaker often comes in handy, especially on coastal runs. On sunny days, hats reduce the fatiguing effects of sun exposure, and in cold weather, they help keep you warm. Sunglasses protect your eyes from the sun as well as from dirt and dust.

Gear and Water Carriers

On longer runs, you may want to carry water and some food. A number of options are available, from lightweight hydration backpacks with a bladder system and mouth hose to lumbar packs that hold water bottles to hand-held water-bottle carriers. Extra pockets in backpacks and lumbar packs will store keys, energy bars, food, and other essentials. Check out what is on the market and decide what your needs are and how much you want to spend.

For further information on equipment, training, and injuries, check out a book devoted to those topics. An excellent one is *The Ultimate Guide to Trail Running: Everything You Need to Know About Equipment, Finding Trails, Nutrition, Hill Strategy, Racing, Training, Weather, First Aid, and Much More*, by Adam W. Chase and Nancy Hobbs.

TRAIL TIPS

- Dress appropriately. Wear layered clothing to be prepared for changeable weather conditions.
- Many trailheads and trails do not have any water sources. Don't drink directly from streams or lakes in the Bay Area, not even water-district reservoirs. The water is not treated and may contain *giardia,* a protozoan that causes severe intestinal illness and discomfort.
- Always carry your own water or sports drink on longer runs and on hot days, and leave some in the car for afterwards. You may also want to carry food on long runs. Energy bars and sports gels are compact and lightweight nourishment, but some runners prefer "real" food like fruit, gorp, or bagels. Experiment a little to find out how your body responds to food and drink while running.
- For a long-distance run, consider toting a first-aid kit in your waist-pack or backpack.
- A cell phone could come in handy on the trail in the case of a sprained ankle or wrong turn.

TRAIL SAFETY

Although most Bay Area parks, preserves, and open-space areas are well traveled by other recreationists, your personal safety should be foremost in your mind. Remember these general guidelines:

- Always carry identification. Write your name, phone number, and blood type on your running shoe. Include important medical information.
- Always let someone know where you are going and what your

route is, even if you just leave a note at home. Run with a partner whenever you can.

- Avoid deserted parks and trails. Trust your intuition and do not continue a run if a person, place, or situation makes you uncomfortable.
- Be alert to your surroundings—to hazards and obstacles on the trail as well as to other people.
- Don't run with headphones. Your hearing is integral to your awareness of surroundings and potential risks.
- Use discretion in acknowledging strangers; ignore verbal harassment and keep moving.
- A small, light canister of pepper spray is a potentially useful item.

TRAIL ETIQUETTE

The Natural Environment

As a trail runner, be aware of your impact on the natural environment and on other trail users. Here are some things to keep in mind:
- Respect the natural habitat—both plants and animals. Do not feed or chase wildlife, tromp on or pick flowers or plants.
- Stay on trails to prevent erosion as well as to avoid poison oak, stinging nettle, and ticks. Avoid areas that are closed for erosion control or revegetation.
- Don't cut switchbacks or make shortcuts. Don't create new trails to avoid muddy sections.
- Pack out your trash. Leave no trace!

Sudden Oak Death

The Sudden Oak Death fungus is killing tanbark oak, coast live oak, black oak, and Shreve's oak in several California counties (Marin, Sonoma, Napa, San Mateo, Santa Cruz, Monterey, Santa Clara, and Alameda). It also has been found on huckleberry, bay laurel, madrone, and rhododendron.

To help prevent the spread of Sudden Oak Death, take the following precautions (adapted from the California Oak Mortality Task Force):
- Park in designated parking areas.
- Stay on established trails and respect trail closures.
- Avoid muddy areas.
- Do not collect wood, acorns, plants, or soil.
- Clean soil and mud off shoes, pets' paws, and car wheels and undercarriage at the nearest gas station.

For more information, visit www.suddenoakdeath.org.

Sharing the Trail

- When you encounter other runners or walkers coming the opposite direction on a narrow trail, step to the right to let them pass.
- When passing other runners or walkers from behind, call out "on your left," to let them know you are behind them and that you intend to pass. Let them know if more runners are behind you.
- On singletracks, when you hear or see mountain bikes coming, step off the trail as soon as possible to let them pass. On wide trails, stay to one side to allow bikes to get by.
- Horses have the right-of-way. Step to the downhill side and greet the rider so the horse knows you are there; do not touch the animals.

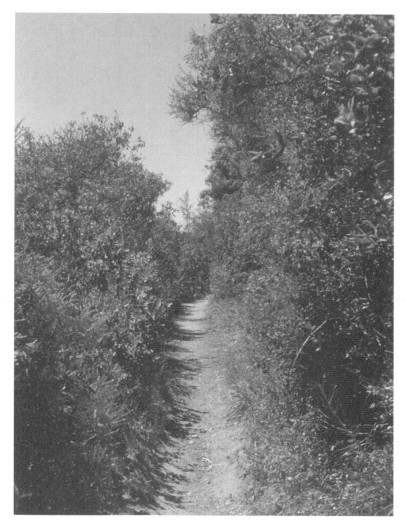

A narrow trail through vegetation on Mt. Tamalpais (Run 19)

- Respect dog regulations. Keep dogs on leash where required. **Dogs** Although the reasons for restrictions may be unclear to you, they are clear to the people who made them. In Point Reyes, for example, dogs are not allowed on most trails because the markings disturb wildlife and interfere with wildlife habitat.
- Don't allow your dogs to chase wildlife.
- Clean up after your dog. Pick up waste in a plastic bag and pack the bag out! Do not leave it on the trail.
- If an unattended dog bothers you on the trail, your best bet is to shout "No!" or "Off!" loudly and authoritatively. A squirt in the face with your water bottle is also a good idea.

HOW TO USE THIS BOOK

Not all of the runs described in this book will work for you. Some will be too long, too steep, or too rocky; some runs may be too short, too flat, or too easy. Note the **Distance** and **Difficulty** ratings, check the **Trail Notes** at the end of each run, and most importantly, read **About the Trail** to find out which runs are for you. Always look at **Alternate Routes** if the featured route isn't appealing. Here is what you can expect from each write-up:

Each route begins with an overview—environment, trails, terrain, exposure, highlights.

Distance: The distance is for the featured route. You'll find alternate route distances under **Alternate Routes**. I have calculated distances to the best of my ability, using the maps and books I refer to in Appendix II. All distances should be considered approximate.

Use: This rating gives you a general idea of how many people you'll see on the featured route. Keep in mind that even at crowded trail-heads and even on weekends, you can almost always find a lightly used route. The rating applies mostly to weekends.

Time: A broad time span for each run reflects differences in pace and style. The times given are based on running 8- and 15-minute miles and then rounded to the nearest quarter of an hour. You may be slower or faster, or may decide to rest or to stop to enjoy a view, but these will give you a general idea of how long the run will take.

Type: Runs in this book are listed as either loop, semi-loop, or out-and-back. A loop means you don't retrace any part of the trail. Semi-loop routes are lollipop-shaped routes that begin and end on the same trail, but include a loop in the middle. Out-and-back runs follow the same trail from the trailhead to the turn-around point and back. Some out-and-back routes can be made into shuttle runs, in which you leave a car at both ends of the route, if you have a willing partner.

High Point/ Low Point: The highest and lowest elevations the route reaches give you a rough idea of how much you'll be climbing and descending. Keep in mind that the route could have either a lot or very few ups and downs within this range. Check the elevation profile for an illustration of the route.

Difficulty: Runs are rated easy, moderate, or strenuous. Difficulty ratings are subjective to a certain degree, but since the ratings in this book are in context with one another, you'll be able to judge the relative difficulty of any trail by comparison with other runs. The ratings take into account the following:
• Steepness: both the intensity of the grade and the number of hills (up and down—sometimes very steep downhills are difficult, too) influence the difficulty rating.
• Distance: longer runs generally are rated more difficult than shorter ones.
• Obstacles: trails with lots of rocks, roots, scree, and eroded sections are harder to run on and receive a higher difficulty rating.

Maps: Many Bay Area parks and recreation areas provide maps at the trailhead. Although usually not topographic, they are useful in helping you follow your route, plot alternate routes, and calculate distances. Check this entry to find out if maps are provided at the trailhead and for other useful maps you can buy. (See also Appendix I.)

Area Management: This is the agency or agencies responsible for the park, preserve, or open-space area where the run is located. Contact them for information about trail closures, conditions, regulations, or other questions or concerns you have. Park officials, rangers, and staff can also be helpful if you need assistance or want to report an incident. (See Appendix I for contact information.)

Map and Elevation Profile: The route maps in this book were created with National Geographic's TOPO! Program and will provide you with a visual depiction of the route, including start- and endpoints, general topography, land features, direction of travel, and elevation loss and gain. The map offers a basic idea of the route; use it in conjunction with a park or preserve map to get a better idea of the area. The elevation profile gives you a rough approximation of the route's highs and lows. Profiles for out-and-back routes are given for one-direction only.

Trailhead Access: This tells you how to reach the trailhead and where to park.

Route Directions: This section only outlines the route and does not describe what the trail is like or what you'll see along the way. It gives you straightforward, unadorned directions—where to turn, which trail to take, which trails you'll pass, and what the distances are.

About the Trail: Read this section before you go to find out the details of the trail—terrain, views, vegetation—described nearly stride-for-stride from a runner's perspective. It will also help acquaint you with some of the plants, trees, and other natural features you will see.

Alternate Routes: If the featured route isn't right for you—or if you want to explore nearby trails—check this section for shorter or longer routes from the same trailhead.

Trail Notes: These bulleted notes provide some additional fast facts about the trail. Check this section to find out:
- What kinds of trails the route includes (fire trail or singletrack)
- What the trail surface is like (rocky, smooth, narrow, wide, muddy, etc.)
- Dog, bike, and horse regulations, so you know if you can bring along your pet and who you'll be sharing the trail with. The listed regulations refer specifically to the trails in the featured run; for general information or restrictions on other trails in the park or preserve, check introductory sections or call the managing agency.
- Toilets, water, and telephone locations

- Day-use fees
- Miscellaneous comments to give you a heads-up about the park or its trails

 Pre-fuel or Re-fuel: The amenities of the city are a short drive from the trailheads in this book. To help you take advantage of them, here are convenient eateries and markets where you can fuel-up with a small snack before your run or enjoy a well-earned feast afterwards.

History

Plants

Geological
features

Wildlife

Nature and History Notes: The more you know about something, the more enjoyable it usually is. In this section you'll find interesting facts about things you'll see on the run.

SAN FRANCISCO AND
MARIN COUNTY TRAIL RUNS

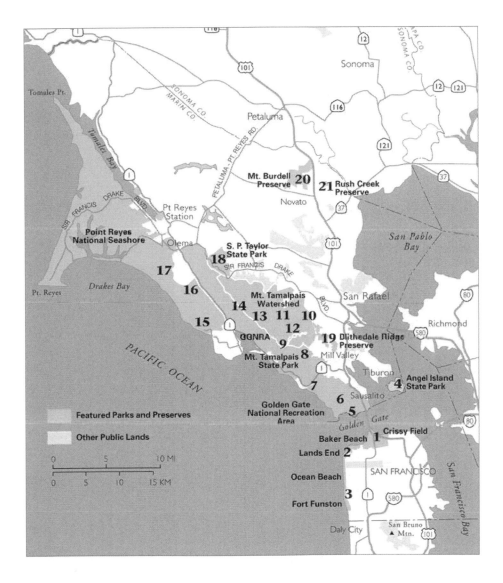

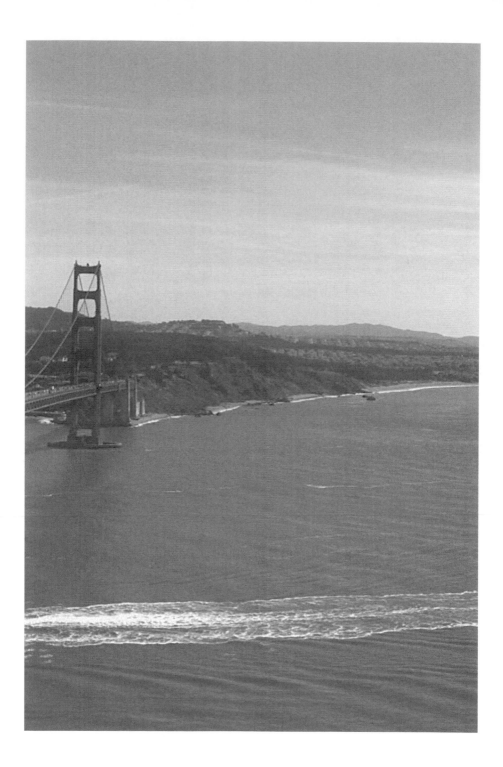

SAN FRANCISCO

LAY OF THE LAND

Celebrated for its cultural attractions, fascinating neighborhoods, and famous landmarks, San Francisco is also reknown for world-class scenery. And not just in the surrounding areas—unlike most urban centers, the city boasts open spaces and national parkland within its city limits.

The unique geography of this region is no small player in its scenic beauty. The city lies at the tip of the San Francisco Peninsula, a long finger of land that forms the western edge of the southern San Francisco Bay. The Santa Cruz Mountains sweep up the peninsula to their northern point just south of San Francisco (San Bruno Mountain). Water surrounds the city on three sides—the Pacific Ocean, the strait of the Golden Gate, and the San Francisco Bay.

Bordering residential San Francisco neighborhoods to the west, Ocean Beach is a 4-mile-long stretch of smooth sand. On clear days, the craggy humps of the Farallon Islands dot the horizon; the islands are part of a national marine sanctuary that extends 12 miles into the ocean from shore. North of the city, the Golden Gate—a mile-wide channel between the bay and the Pacific—separates San Francisco from Marin County and lends its name to the famous bridge. Steep vermilion cliffs on the Marin side match the color of the Golden Gate Bridge. East of San Francisco, the bay extends for 420 square miles—50 miles long and from 1 to 12 miles wide. Alcatraz, Yerba Buena, and Angel islands dot the waters. The East Bay hills, topped by Mt. Diablo, rise in the distance. Testament to the beauty—and social activism—of this City by the Bay, much of San Francisco's bayshore and coastline are protected as part of a 75,000-acre national park, the Golden Gate National Recreation Area.

Although the city is known for its precipitous hills, the San Francisco runs in this book travel the edges of the city's hilly land mass (and one of the bay's islands) and are relatively flat. They explore Ocean Beach, the coastal cliffs at Lands End, the bay shoreline along

Opposite page: View of Baker Beach and the Golden Gate Bridge from the Marin Highlands

Crissy Field, and landmark Angel Island. You can easily schedule these runs into your daily routine, or take a weekend day to discover (or rediscover) these parts of San Francisco. Running is one of the best ways to get to know a city—for locals and visitors alike.

GOLDEN GATE NATIONAL RECREATION AREA

The Golden Gate National Recreation Area is the world's largest urban national park, with 75,398 total acres and 28 miles of coastline. GGNRA land stretches south from San Francisco to Milagra and Sweeney ridges on the peninsula, and north along the Marin Headlands and popular Muir and Stinson beaches to Bolinas Ridge and the San Andreas fault zone in Olema Valley. Diverse plant and animal communities live within this protected area: raptors soar over high ridges searching for prey; lizards sun themselves on rocks and dart across trails; salamanders crawl beneath towering redwoods, where the forest floor is thick with thimbleberry bushes and ferns; and endangered Mission Blue and San Bruno Elfin butterflies rely on silver-leaf lupine and stonecrop in these safe habitats.

Easy access is another of GGNRA's exceptional qualities. For some, GGNRA lands are just beyond their doorstep; for others, they are a short drive from home; and for visitors, the GGNRA's proximity to the cities of the Bay Area make them easily reachable by car or public transportation.

The runs in this book on GGNRA lands include: Ocean Beach, Lands End, Crissy Field, Rodeo Valley, Green Gulch, Gerbode Valley, and Bolinas Ridge. For more information about the GGNRA, see the individual runs.

1

CRISSY FIELD TO BAKER BEACH

A quintessential San Francisco run, this urban trail along the bayshore and coastline of the city offers thrilling views around the bay. You'll enjoy the San Francisco scene with runners, walkers, bicyclists, and dogs along the wide promenade at Crissy Field, and may be lucky enough to happen upon a catamaran or outrigger canoe race. Beyond the Golden Gate Bridge, you follow a narrow path on high coastal bluffs and turn around after a sandy jaunt across Baker Beach.

Distance	6 miles
Time	0.75–1.5 hours
Type	out-and-back
High Point/Low Point	276′/3′
Difficulty	moderate
Use	moderate
Maps	GGNRA map (available at Presidio visitor center, Cliff House visitor center, Warming Hut)
Area Management	Golden Gate National Recreation Area

Trailhead Access

From Hwy. 1, take the Doyle Dr. exit and continue past the Palace of Fine Arts to Marina Blvd. Turn left into the parking lot at the east end of the Golden Gate Promenade. Make a U-turn at the first possible intersection and go west on Marina Blvd. to Baker St. Keep to the right and continue straight into the Presidio on Mason St. Turn right into East Beach parking lot.

From Interstate 80, follow The Embarcadero to Bay St. Turn left on Bay and continue past Fort Mason to Marina Blvd. Veer right on Marina Blvd. and follow it to its end at the Baker St. Keep to the right and continue straight into the Presidio on Mason St. Turn right into East Beach parking lot.

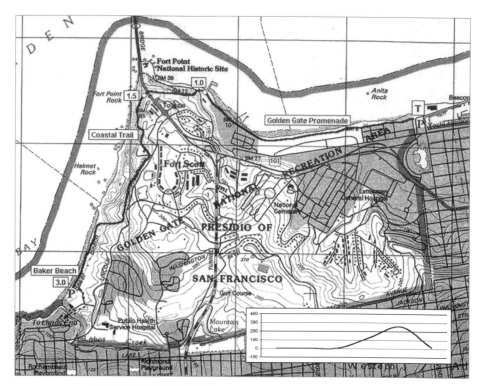

CRISSY FIELD TO BAKER BEACH

Route Directions Pick up the shoreline **Golden Gate Promenade/San Francisco Bay Trail** just beyond the parking lot.

1.0 Veer left just beyond Crissy Field Warming Hut to meet Fort Point Rd. (Follow signs to Golden Gate Bridge.)

1.2 Climb wooden staircase signed to GOLDEN GATE BRIDGE.

1.3 Turn right at top of stairs; follow trail through low tunnel.

1.4 Veer left at fork; cross under Golden Gate Bridge.

1.5 Turn right on **Coastal Trail**. Follow signs for Bay Area Ridge Trail.

1.8 Veer right to stay on Coastal Trail.

2.3 Veer left toward Lincoln Dr. Follow roadside path along Lincoln Dr.

2.6 Veer right to continue on Coastal Trail to Baker Beach.

2.8 Rejoin pavement at far end of parking lot.

3.0 Turn-around point. Retrace your steps.

Begin this route by heading east along the graveled Golden Gate Promenade, between East Beach and Crissy Field. A recent restoration project has converted Crissy Field from an asphalt expanse surrounded by a chain link fence to the thriving marshland it once was. Pickleweed, cordgrass, cow clover, saltmarsh arrow, and other native plants grace the shoreline dunes; look for birds in the newly restored tidal marsh. Expansive views of the Bay Area surround you: the red cliffs of the Marin Headlands across the Golden Gate; Angel Island, which looks like land from your vantage point; Alcatraz rising in the foreground of the East Bay hills; and the colorful sails of windsurfers and sailboats crowding the bay in fair weather.

You pass the Gulf of the Farallones National Marine Sanctuary visitor center, the Historic Coast Guard Station, and the Crissy Field Warming Hut, which houses a café and bookstore. Veer left just beyond the hut, following signs to the Golden Gate Bridge. Cross the road to Fort Point and look for a wooden staircase signed to the Golden Gate Bridge.

You'll see evidence of a habitat restoration project underway, in which the National Park Service is removing the non-native eucalyptus trees that grow throughout the Presidio. At the top of the staircase, a dirt path leads through a low brick tunnel (watch your head) and emerges at a scenic picnic site. From here you have your first views of the bridge at eye level. Just beyond, you join the narrow Coastal Trail, which traces the bluffs on loose, sandy dirt. Lupine, ceanothus, and other coastal scrub plants line the trail.

When the coast is cloaked in fog, you'll feel like you're on the edge of a mystical world. On clear days, the views are spectacular: the rugged San Francisco bluffs stretch to Lands End, where they drop steeply to rocky coves. Across the Golden Gate, the rust-colored hills of the Marin Headlands rise steeply from the water. Point Bonita juts west into the Pacific, and a lighthouse on the tip warns boats of their proximity to the often fog-masked shoreline.

Following signs for the Bay Area Ridge Trail, you climb a set of wooden stairs and pass two defunct Coastal Defense Batteries, built in the late 1800s. Bypassing signs for the Ridge Trail where it heads left into the Presidio, you continue across a gravel parking area to the singletrack Coastal Trail. You soon find yourself next to Lincoln Drive on a narrow path that hugs the road and descends gradually. Be careful to avoid the clumps of poison oak that hem the trail. Shortly before the bottom of the hill, the roadside path ends at a

About the Trail

For an up-close view of the bay and bridge, continue a quarter of a mile on the road to Fort Point (paved, but well worth the trip). On windy days, waves sometimes wash over the pavement along this stretch of road. Follow the road to the back side of the fort for a fish-eye view of the massive bridge. Then retrace your steps to the wooden staircase that climbs to the bridge. On your way, take in the splendid views of Coit Tower, Alcatraz, Angel Island, and the East Bay.

chain-link fence and you head right toward Baker Beach on a wide, gravel road. On a short sprint across the sand, you'll have views west to the craggy cliffs of Lands End. The end of Baker Beach is a good place to turn around, or you can continue on to Lands End (see Alternate Routes).

Alternate Routes This run combines well with the Lands End route (see Run 2) for about a 12-mile out-and-back or a 6-mile shuttle trip. Follow the description of the featured run to Baker Beach. From the far (west) end of the Baker Beach parking lot, pick up a small sandy dirt path next to the Presidio Water Treatment Plant and follow it back out to Lincoln Blvd. (called El Camino del Mar here). Turn right on the sidewalk and then right again on 26th Avenue. Turn left on Seacliff Avenue and follow it to where it rejoins El Camino del Mar, part of the 49-mile Scenic Drive. The Lands End section of the Coastal Trail begins 1.2 miles from Baker Beach.

Trail Notes • Wide promenade, stairs, and singletrack
• Some roots on narrow Coastal Trail; parts of Coastal Trail sandy; on sand at Baker Beach
• Dogs on leash
• Bikes on Golden Gate Promenade along Crissy Field
• Horses allowed
• Toilet at trailhead, Warming Hut, Golden Gate Bridge parking lot (short detour from route), Fort Point, and Baker Beach
• Water at trailhead and Baker Beach
• No fees
• This is a popular route, especially along Crissy Field and near the bridge. You'll find more solitude on the Coastal Trail.

 Overlooking the marsh, the Crissy Field Center Café is a great spot to get a light breakfast or lunch. The center runs an innovative environmental outreach program, which includes field classes about arctic birds, natural sound recording, wetland ecology, and whale-watching. The center also has a small bookstore and provides information about Crissy Field and the GGNRA. Open Wednesday through Sunday, 9 AM to 5 PM

The Embarcadero Farmer's Market is a lively place to buy fresh fruit, veggies, and breads before or after a run. You'll find it on Saturdays at Embarcadero and Green Street (8 AM to 1 PM) and on

Tuesdays at Embarcadero and Market Street in Justin Herman Plaza (10:30 AM to 2:30 PM).

In stark contrast to the thriving tidal marsh and dunes at Crissy Field today, a paved military airstrip covered the bayshore here for most of the 20th century. In 1998, the National Park Service began an ambitious project to restore the natural ecosystem. The project entailed a massive effort on the part of skilled engineers and volunteers. During the years of military use, more than 87,000 tons of hazardous material had accumulated. This material was removed, and another 70 acres of asphalt and concrete were removed and recycled as foundation material for newly created pathways and parking lots. More than 200,000 cubic yards of soil were dug up to restore the tidal marsh, and 15,000 tons of rubble were cleaned up along the shoreline. Finally, volunteers spent more than 2,400 hours planting and maintaining 100,000 plants, representing 73 native species. The 20-acre tidal marsh at Crissy Field now attracts native wildlife, such as bay shrimp, Dungeness crabs, great blue herons, peregrine falcons, and red-tailed hawks.

Nature Notes

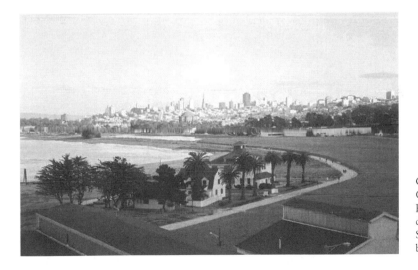

Crissy Field and Golden Gate Promenade with downtown San Francisco beyond

2

LANDS END TRAIL

Hanging precariously on the cliffs of Point Lobos, this path is one of San Francisco's treasures. Come prepared for the fog that envelopes these windswept coastal cliffs. Clear days bring remarkable vistas of the Golden Gate Bridge, Mt. Tamalpais, and the Marin Headlands. The trail is a wide, smooth, and sandy path. It is fairly level, with the exception of one staircase climb that gets your heart pumping.

Distance	3.4 miles
Time	0.5-1 hour
Type	out-and-back
High Point/Low Point	310´/132´
Difficulty	easy
Use	moderate
Maps	GGNRA map (available at Presidio visitor center, Cliff House visitor center, Warming Hut)
Area Management	Golden Gate National Recreation Area

Trailhead Access From Hwy. 1 northbound, turn left on Geary Blvd. Turn right on 25th Ave. and then left on El Camino del Mar (Lincoln Blvd. goes right). Continue to just past 32nd Ave. and park on the street. Trailhead is on the right side of the street.

From Hwy. 1 southbound, exit on Lincoln Blvd. and follow it until it becomes El Camino del Mar. Continue to just past 32nd Ave. and park on the street. Trailhead is on the right side of the street.

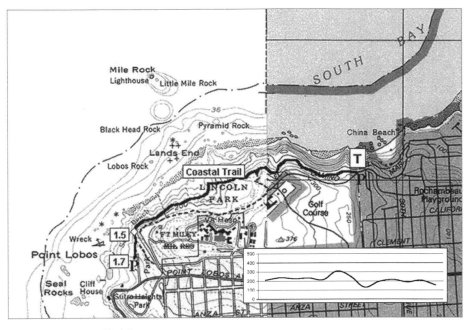

LAND'S END TRAIL

Begin on El Camino del Mar at LANDS END sign.

Route Directions

1.5 Veer right on wide trail.

1.7 Merrie Way parking lot. Retrace route to trailhead.

This run is on a mostly smooth, sandy dirt path, with only the occasional intrusion of a rock or Monterey cypress root. Shortly after starting out, you reach a wooden lookout point. Pause here to take in impressive views east toward the Golden Gate Bridge, an unusual perspective on the entryway to the bay. A few steps beyond, your view expands to include the small stretch of sand at Baker Beach and the protected cove of China Beach. On clear days, you'll see across the Golden Gate to the Marin Headlands, where Point Bonita lighthouse sits at the tip of the land.

About the Trail

The trail narrows as ceanothus, twinberry honeysuckle, and (avoidable) poison oak crowd its edges. Climb the route's single hill on wooden steps placed in the deep sand and immediately descend a staircase on the other side. The path widens again, lined by wind-contoured Monterey cypress and pine trees. Through the branches you catch glimpses of Mile Rock just off the coast, where many a ship has run aground. From the turnaround point at the Merrie Way parking lot, you'll see the Cliff House perched on the cliff edge, as its name indicates; if you jog across the parking lot you'll catch a glimpse of the famous old Sutro Baths landmark just below you.

Alternate Routes If you begin from the Merrie Way parking lot, you can extend this route by continuing on to Baker Beach, the Golden Gate Bridge, or Crissy Field. From Merrie Way it is 2.8 miles to Baker Beach, 4.3 to the Golden Gate Bridge, and 5.8 to Crissy Field. You must cross through the residential Seacliff neighborhood to reach Baker Beach:
At the end of the Lands End trail, turn left on El Camino del Mar.
Veer left on Seacliff Avenue.
Turn right on 26th Avenue.
Turn left on El Camino del Mar.
Turn left on the first dirt path at the bottom of the hill.
Run through Monterey pines to Baker Beach.
Follow Run 1, Crissy Field to Baker Beach, in reverse from here.

Trail Notes • Singletrack and wide trails; stairs
• Sandy dirt; some small rocks
• No bikes
• Dogs on leash
• Horses allowed
• Bathroom and phone at GGNRA Cliff House visitor center
• No fees
• WARNING: the cliffs at Lands End are steep, rapidly eroding, and precarious; respect the signs and do not climb on the cliffs.
• You'll encounter runners, walkers, and tourists on this popular trail.

Try family-owned Louis' restaurant, just west of the parking lot on Merrie Way, for juicy burgers and thick milkshakes. Further east on Clement Street, you'll find plenty of other options: cafes, delicatessens, small markets, and Japanese, Thai, and Korean restaurants.

History Notes The Lands End trail follows the route of an old steam railroad that once ran along these cliffs. The easily eroded, unstable land was prone to landslides, which forced the abandonment of the railroad.

3

OCEAN BEACH TO
FORT FUNSTON

Beaches in San Francisco? It may not compare to those in Hawaii or San Diego, but Ocean Beach is San Francisco's very own stretch of sandy Pacific coastline. This western edge of the city is often blustery and ensconced in fog—perfect trail running conditions. Follow the beach for up to 4 miles; if you choose to do a shuttle trip, you can climb the coastal cliffs at Fort Funston and run along a paved path to reach your car. High tide may limit the length of this run when it covers the beach.

Distance	4.7 miles one way; up to 9.4 miles
Time	up to 2.25 hours
Type	shuttle or out-and-back
High Point/Low Point	149′/1′
Difficulty	easy to moderate
Use	light
Maps	GGNRA map (available at Presidio visitor center, Cliff House visitor center, Warming Hut)
Area Management	Golden Gate National Recreation Area

North trailhead From Hwy. 1, go west on Geary Blvd. Veer right on Point Lobos Ave. and follow it past the Cliff House to the Great Highway. Turn right to park in the lot at Balboa St. and the Great Highway.

South trailhead From Skyline Blvd. (Hwy. 35), go 0.1 mile past John Muir Dr. and turn right into Fort Funston. Bear right at the fork and continue to the parking lot. (Northbound travelers on Skyline Blvd. should make a U-turn at John Muir Dr. and follow directions above.)

Trailhead Access

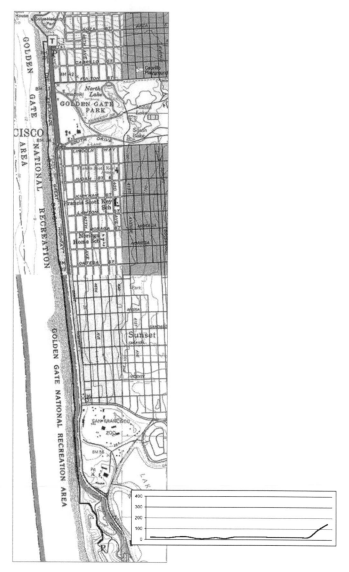

OCEAN BEACH TO FORT FUNSTON

Route Directions

Begin at far north end of Ocean Beach

1.1 Lincoln Way

3.1 San Francisco Zoo.

4.0 Beach below Fort Funston.

4.7 Fort Funston parking area.

From the parking area at the north trailhead (Balboa Street and the Great Highway), enter the beach by way of one of several stairwells from the sidewalk. Four miles of flat, smooth sand lie before you, bordered to the west by the Pacific Ocean and to the east by the 3-mile paved trail along the Great Highway. The sea wall and esplanade separating the beach from the road were built in 1929.

Continue as far as you like. Though you may not be able to cross the rocks that splay across the sand west of the zoo (if the tide is high), the most picturesque part of this run is the beach below the high, eroding cliffs of Fort Funston. You'll see evidence of the landslides that send parts of these unstable sandstone cliffs (and sometimes the house built atop them) into the Pacific with winter storms. Several use-paths climb the cliffs to the dunes above and eventually lead to Fort Funston. If the day is free of fog, you'll see south down the coast to Mussel Rock, the point where the San Andreas fault leaves the ocean and enters land, and beyond to San Pedro Point in Pacifica.

If you do continue to Fort Funston, from the viewing deck watch for colorful hang gliders riding on ocean breezes.

Alternate Routes

To begin or end this run at another location, park at one of several points along the Great Highway—across from Golden Gate Park; at Sloat Blvd.; or south of Sloat Blvd., shortly before the junction of Skyline Blvd. and the Great Highway.

Head into Golden Gate Park (between Fulton Street and Lincoln Way) to combine this sandy route with forested park paths.

Trail Notes

• Sand
• Dogs on leash
• No bikes
• Horses allowed
• Bathroom and phone at GGNRA Cliff House visitor center and at Fort Funston
• No fees
• At high tide, you may have difficulty getting around a jumble of shoreline rocks where Sloat Blvd. meets the Great Highway.

WARNING: Strong currents, riptides, and heavy surf make swimming and wading at Ocean Beach dangerous and inadvisable.

At the end of your run, recuperate at the Beach Chalet, at the tip of Golden Gate Park and just across the Great Highway from Ocean Beach. Designed by Willis Polk in 1925, the Beach Chalet doubles as a visitor center and a restaurant/brewery. On the ground floor, Works Progress Administration (WPA) murals, woodcarvings, and mosaics portray scenes of Depression-era San Francisco. Upstairs, the restaurant offers decadent Saturday and Sunday brunches, bistro-style cuisine, and house-made ales—plus great views of the Pacific!

History Notes

Before early San Franciscans developed these outlying areas of the city, great sand dunes stretched inland from the Pacific Coast. Initial attempts to create Golden Gate Park were met with little faith that even a blade of grass would grow in the shifting sand. Today, the 1017-acre, lavishly vegetated park and the row houses of the Sunset district cover the dunes, and virtually nothing remains of the city's sandy past.

4

ANGEL ISLAND

Run in circles in the bay, with round-the-bay panoramic views. Angel Island offers cool breezes off the water, forested hillsides, a fun ferry ride, and both narrow singletrack trails and wide fire roads. It's an ideal excursion for a trail run.

Distance	8.2 miles
Time	1–2 hours
Type	loop
High Point/Low Point	781´/56´
Difficulty	easy–moderate
Use	light
Maps	State park map $1 from kiosk at boat dock
Area Management	California State Parks

Trailhead Access

Catch the ferry to Angel Island from Tiburon (415) 435-2131; Alameda or Oakland (510) 522-3300; San Francisco (415) 773-1188; or Vallejo (707) 64-FERRY or (877) 64-FERRY.

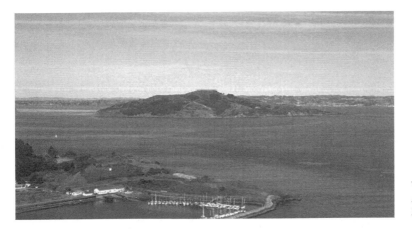

View of Angel Island from Marin Headlands

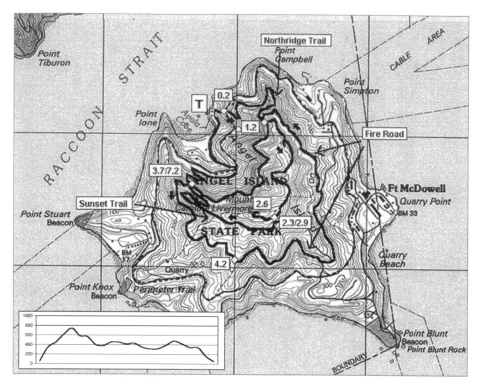

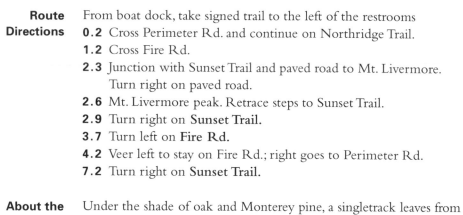

ANGEL ISLAND

**Route
Directions**

From boat dock, take signed trail to the left of the restrooms

0.2 Cross Perimeter Rd. and continue on Northridge Trail.

1.2 Cross Fire Rd.

2.3 Junction with Sunset Trail and paved road to Mt. Livermore. Turn right on paved road.

2.6 Mt. Livermore peak. Retrace steps to Sunset Trail.

2.9 Turn right on **Sunset Trail.**

3.7 Turn left on **Fire Rd.**

4.2 Veer left to stay on Fire Rd.; right goes to Perimeter Rd.

7.2 Turn right on **Sunset Trail.**

**About the
Trail**

Under the shade of oak and Monterey pine, a singletrack leaves from the boat dock area (signed to the NORTHRIDGE TRAIL, PERIMETER ROAD, AND MT. LIVERMORE) and immediately climbs a steep grade, with no opportunity for a warm-up. After a long series of steps, you meet the paved Perimeter Road. Take in views of Marin County here—west to the Tiburon peninsula, Mt. Tamalpais, and coastal ridges. Continue across Perimeter Road on the Northridge Trail, now a gradual singletrack through a light forest of oak, bay laurel, and tree-size ceanothus. In spring, blue ceanothus flowers cast their strong fragrance over the trail, and California poppies, blue dicks, blue-eyed grass, and morning glory bloom in open stretches. Beneath oak and bay laurel trees, leaf duff covers the trail as it continues a gradual uphill on long switchbacks; hazelnut, blackberry, and honeysuckle grow in the understory.

As you gain elevation, the trail becomes rockier and reaches exposed, drier terrain, where manzanita grows in sandy soil. Just past the one-mile point, your trail crosses the broad dirt Fire Road. You stay on the Northridge Trail, which wraps around the northeast side of the island. You enter forest again and have tree-screened views of the East Bay. Gooseberry, currant, and snowberry grow beneath oaks along the leaf-covered trail, dangling deep purple or white berries in fall and winter.

The trail emerges on an open grassy plateau that is covered with yarrow, wild iris, and checkerbloom in spring. Manzanita predominates along this level stretch, joined by coyote bush, ceanothus, and stands of cascading bunchgrasses. Here you have your first views of Mt. Livermore ahead. After a couple of brief climbs, your trail ends at a paved road, and the Sunset Trail begins just across it. Turn right on the road, a straight-shot to the top of 781-foot Mt. Livermore on a steep but brief grind. Pause long enough on the peak to take in the 360-degree views around the bay (signposts tell you what you're seeing and how far away the landmarks are—Mt. Tam is 9 miles, Crissy Field 4 miles, and the Golden Gate Bridge 5 miles) before retracing your steps down the paved road to the Sunset Trail.

Head west on the Sunset Trail toward the Golden Gate, the broad waterway into the bay, flanked by the sparkling buildings of San Francisco to the south and the coastal ridges of Marin County to the north. In the 1800s, the military planted eucalyptus trees on these hillsides, but in recent years the state park has cut most of the trees to allow native shrubs and grasses to recover. The nearly level trail now crosses open grasslands sprinkled with coyote bush and poison oak, and in spring, the site of many wildflowers.

Turn left on the Fire Road where it intersects the Sunset Trail. (You will loop back to this point and finish the run on the lower part of the Sunset Trail.) The wide, smooth Fire Road trail circles the island at an elevation of about 400 feet, on a mostly level route. You return to views of the East Bay as you head east on the trail and cross the same exposed slopes as you traversed on the Sunset Trail. As you wrap around the island, follow signs for the Fire Road at each junction, also signed as the BIKE ROUTE. You'll pass a couple of cut-offs to Mt. Livermore, a turn-off to Perimeter Road, and a road to the Immigration Station, where your trail makes a sharp left and climbs briefly to pass a water station.

As you round the east and north sides of the island, oak, buckeye, madrone, and tree-size toyon bushes, heavy with red berries in fall and winter, shade the trail. You have views of the East Bay hills as they slope toward sea level in Richmond, as well as views of the Richmond-San Rafael Bridge, Tiburon, and Belvedere.

Back at your starting point on the Fire Road, you turn left on the continuation of the Sunset Trail, marked only with a no bikes sign. The narrow trail descends through a cool forest on long, gradual switchbacks. You meet Perimeter Road and cross it to join a paved road from Ayala Cove. Continue beneath tall eucalyptus to Ayala Cove, past the visitor center and picnic areas, to the boat dock.

Alternate Routes
Angel Island offers 12 miles of trails and a surprising number of routes within its relatively small acreage. For an easy run, the dirt Fire Road makes an almost completely flat loop around the island. For a slightly longer loop with a few hills, circle the island on the paved Perimeter Road. Combine the Northridge and Sunset trails for a shorter loop (about 4.5 miles) on the island's two singletrack trails.

Trail Notes
- Singletrack and fire trails
- Generally smooth trails; a few rocky sections on Northridge and Sunset trails
- No dogs
- Bikes allowed on Perimeter and Fire roads
- No horses
- Restrooms at boat dock and Ayala Cove
- Water at boat dock

 A café at the boat dock on the island serves snacks during the summer months. The rest of the year, vending machines are your only option on the island.

In Tiburon, a row of restaurants and cafes along the waterfront offer full meals, brunch, pizza, deli sandwiches, and baked goods. Many have outdoor seating with great views of Angel Island. You'll find two grocery stores on the main drag, a few blocks from the waterfront.

In 1910, after half a century of military presence on Angel Island, the federal government opened an Immigration Station. Over the next 30 years, the station received mostly Asian immigrants; about 175,000 Chinese had entered the United States via Angel Island before the station was closed in 1940. **History Notes**

Unlike Ellis Island, the purpose of the Immigration Station at Angel Island was primarily to keep new arrivals out of the country. Most immigrants were detained on the island for two weeks to six months while their cases were being decided. Some, however, were kept there for up to two years waiting to hear if they would be deported or allowed to stay in the country. The wooden walls of the dormitories, where some detainees carved their thoughts in poetry, record their frustration with their situation.

After the bombing of Pearl Harbor in 1941, the Immigration Station was turned into processing facility for prisoners of war; hundreds of Japanese and German prisoners were held on the island. Today, the old barracks building is a museum where visitors can view a recreated dormitory and some of the remaining wall poetry.

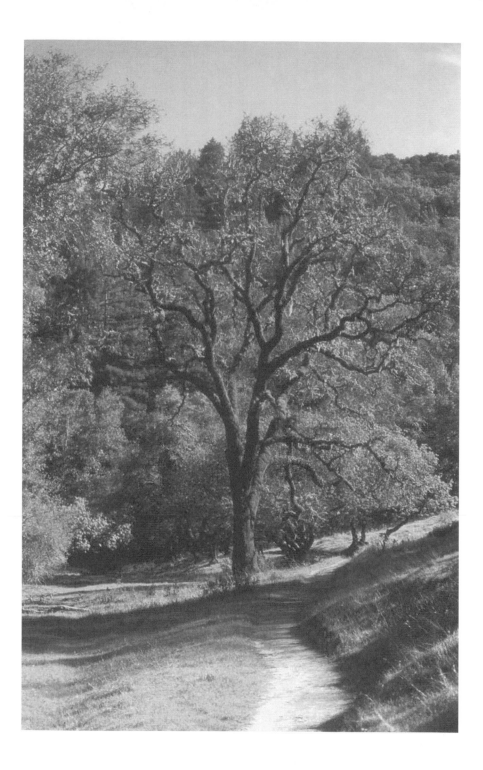

MARIN COUNTY

LAY OF THE LAND

Comprised of the land north of the bay, Marin County is perhaps the Bay Area's best known outdoor recreation region. The county is home to vibrant variations in coastal and inland landscape, vegetation, and climate. Marin's high points—Barnabe Mountain, Mt. Tamalpais, and Mt. Burdell—offer a clear view of the lay of the land, from coastal ridges to inland valleys to bayside wetlands.

Just north of the Golden Gate, the rolling hills of the Marin Headlands meet the coast at dramatic cliffs and rugged beaches. Trails in the headlands are popular since they are convenient to many Bay Area locations—adjacent to Marin towns and a short drive from San Francisco and the East Bay. North of the headlands, steep slopes rise from the coast at Stinson Beach to meet grasslands and redwood forests on the western side of Mt. Tamalpais.

Mt. Tam, as it is often called, dominates Marin's landscape. It spans the county's coastal and inland areas and encompasses climate and vegetation zones from each. Exposed coastal grasslands yield to oak woodland, chaparral, redwood forest, and riparian enclaves on eastern, northern, and southern faces. The mountain's slopes ease into neighborhoods on its east side and provide convenient access to residents and visitors.

Bolinas Ridge descends from the northern slopes of Mt. Tamalpais and bridges Olema Valley to the west and Samuel P. Taylor State Park to the east. The San Andreas fault cuts through Olema Valley, a straight line between Bolinas Lagoon in the south and Tomales Bay in the north. West of the valley, the Point Reyes peninsula juts into the Pacific; on this unique cape, smooth coastal beaches meet rocky cliffs and forested ridges give way to pastoral inland valleys. Each of Point Reyes' distinct landscapes is remarkable, each well worth the trip to this outlying national seashore, just an hour or so's drive from San Francisco or the East Bay.

East of Point Reyes, grassy slopes extend from creekside redwood

Opposite page: Oak tree on Hidden Meadow Trail at Phoenix Lake

57

forests in Samuel P. Taylor State Park, and rise to 1466-foot Barnabe Mountain. Oak woodlands cover inland valleys, where temperatures are more extreme than on the coast. Northeast of San Francisco Bay, Mt. Burdell crowns Marin's interior at 1558 feet. Just east of Mt. Burdell, wetlands like those at Rush Creek thrive along the Petaluma River, on its course to San Pablo Bay.

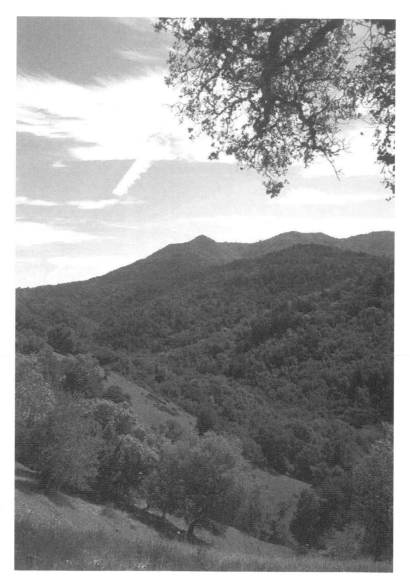

View of
Mt Tamalpais
from the
Yolanda Trail
(Run 10)

MARIN HEADLANDS

A spectacular series of coastal ridges stretches north from the Golden Gate. Known as the Marin Headlands, these 10,000 acres of open space drop steeply to the ocean, where the Pacific crashes onto rugged beaches. The hills roll inland, golden brown in summer and fall, and glistening green in winter and spring, when they come alive with richly colored wildflowers. The ridges' high points offer panoramic views of the Bay Area.

Until the Golden Gate National Recreation Area acquired this area in 1972, the U.S. Army occupied the southern headlands. The army constructed artillery batteries and forts that were used in the early 1900s and during WWII; in the 1950s it built Nike missile sites on the headlands. An unintended consequence of the army's presence was to prevent development of these desirable lands, which were coveted for their scenic location and their convenience to San Francisco.

The northern valleys of the headlands, populated by Portuguese dairy ranches, were not thus protected from developers' voracious plans, and the construction of the Golden Gate Bridge and rapid post-WWII growth turned the valleys into the targets of urban development schemes. Plans for Marincello, a 2138-acre community of homes, shopping malls, hotels, and highrises outraged devoted conservationists, who launched a fierce battle to preserve the land as open space. Martha Gerbode, a San Francisco environmentalist, provided money to the Nature Conservancy to buy the land, and the conservancy then turned it over to the park service. The area once slated for development is now named Gerbode Valley.

The weather at the Marin Headlands varies dramatically. On some days white wisps of fog filter over the ridges, offering protection from the sun's heat but not obscuring coastal views. On other days you can't see the hillside in front of you for thick fog. The exposed trails here offer no protection from sun, wind, or fog. Come prepared with a hat, windbreaker, and sunscreen.

What You'll Find

There are several trailheads in the Marin Headlands. The three headlands runs in this book start from the Golden Gate Bridge and the Tennessee Valley trailheads. The Golden Gate National Recreation visitor center on Bunker Road in Rodeo Valley, open daily from 9:30 am to 4:30 pm, staffs rangers who can answer questions about trails in the headlands; you'll also find maps and information about dog regulations.

5

RODEO VALLEY LOOP

Outstanding views of San Francisco and the surrounding coastline are the highlights of this route. The trailhead is the north end of the Golden Gate Bridge. You'll climb a singletrack path to a high ridge and dip into the broad lowland of Rodeo Valley, where wide trails lead up the valley and back to the ridgeline above Sausalito.

Distance	7.3 miles
Time	1–1.75 hours
Type	semi-loop
High Point/Low Point	884'/95'
Difficulty	moderate
Use	light
Maps	GGNRA map
	available at visitor center)
Area Management	Golden Gate National Recreation Area

Trailhead Access From Hwy. 101 northbound, take the Alexander Ave. exit, turn left, and go under the highway. Turn right on Conzelman Rd. and make an immediate left on the first road, to the bridge parking lot.

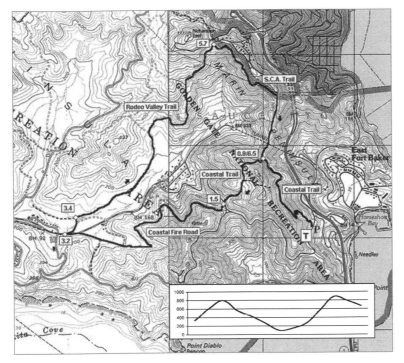

RODEO VALLEY LOOP

NOTE: The mileage posted at the trailhead is wrong—actual distance to Rodeo Beach is 4.2 miles.

Begin on the **Coastal Trail** at north end of parking lot.

Route Directions

0.1 Cross Conzelman Rd.

0.8 Turn left on junction with **SCA Trail** to continue on Coastal Trail.

1.2 Pass side trail on left.

1.5 Cross McCullogh Rd. Join **Coastal Fire Rd.** at gravel parking area.

3.0 Go around white metal gate.

3.1 Pass Coastal Trail offshoot on left.

3.2 Cross Bunker Rd. in crosswalk to dirt parking area.

3.3 Cross service road to Rodeo Valley Trail signpost. Cross wooden bridge and turn right on **Rodeo Valley Trail.**

3.4 Turn right again on Rodeo Valley Trail.

5.7 Turn right on **SCA Trail.**

6.5 Turn left on Coastal Trail.

About the Trail Start off on the singletrack trail at the north end of the parking area. Just below you, the massive Golden Gate Bridge crosses the mile-wide waterway between the bay and ocean. The trail emerges from a small grove of Monterey cypress and climbs through a thicket of coyote bush and sagebrush to cross Conzelman Road. Signs here and throughout this route remind you that this is Mission Blue butterfly habitat—the silver-leaved lupine that grow on these coastal hills is a host plant for the endangered butterfly and vital to the butterfly's survival. Wooden posts strung with thick metal cord intermittently mark the edges of the trail to protect the vegetation.

Switchbacks make for a moderate climb up the steep ridge. Highway 101 roars below you on this first part of the route. Lupine, coyote bush, coffeeberry, grasses, and an occasional sculpted oak line the narrow trail. Views abound, so keep one eye out for rocks in the trail and the other eye on the stunning panorama of the Golden Gate Bridge, San Francisco, Angel Island, and the East Bay.

Just before the ridge, you meet the SCA (Student Conservation Association) Trail, your return route. Stay to the left on the Coastal Trail and make a last spurt to the ridgetop along the narrow, rocky path. A muted mosaic of vegetation and rock outcroppings in green, grey, and brown stretches to the Pacific, across broad Rodeo Valley to Rodeo Beach. Your trail widens and descends west on gravelly, decomposing red chert (see **Nature Notes** below). Between dips in the ridge to the south, you see the wide strait of the Golden Gate west of the bridge and the rugged cliffs of San Francisco's Lands End; to the north, Wolf Ridge rises severely between Rodeo and Tennessee valleys; ahead, you can trace your route, cut into the folded, russet-colored, chert walls of the hillside.

Cross McCullough Road and continue through a parking area and around a metal gate. The wide, gravelly Coastal Fire Road hugs the hillside as it descends into the valley; the cluster of houses on the floor along Bunker Road were formerly used by the military. The trail levels near the road and you go around another metal gate, skirt a grassy field, and pass an offshoot of the Coastal Trail.

Across Bunker Road and beyond another gravel parking area, you join the Rodeo Valley Trail and begin the second half of this loop. The wide, grassy trail heads east, toward the high ridge that rings the valley. Willows, reeds, and rushes thrive in the moist soil along the creekbed that initially borders the trail. During wet weather, this section of the route may be boggy. In spring, blue lupine blossoms adorn low bushes; bright yellow suncups and coast sunflower decorate hillsides of coffeeberry, sagebrush, blackberry, and coyote bush; and orange-red Indian paintbrush grows on rocky trail cuts. Opulent exposures of red chert paint the hillsides across Bunker Road.

As you climb higher toward the ridge, you look down on Rodeo Valley, divided by Bunker Road, with the Pacific Ocean beyond. Private homes dot the ridgetop above. After a couple of miles of gradual uphill, you reach the crest and turn on the SCA Trail. This smooth singletrack curves around the head of the valley, hugging the hillside just below the ridgecrest. You have breathtaking views of the Golden Gate Bridge with San Francisco beyond, and of the Santa Cruz Mountains as they travel south down the peninsula, flanked by the ocean and the bay. Westerly views take in the Pacific beyond the headlands, with the Rodeo Valley Trail in the foreground. The trail begins a gentle but rocky descent to meet the Coastal Trail, on which you retrace your steps to the Golden Gate Bridge.

Alternate Routes

Combine this run with one from the Tennessee Valley Trailhead (see Runs 6 and 7) for a long "tour de headlands." From the junction with the Rodeo Valley Trail just past Bunker Road, turn left and continue to the Miwok Trail. Climb to Wolf Ridge on the Miwok Trail and dip into Tennessee Valley or continue on the ridgetop to the Bobcat Trail. You can pick up the SCA Trail via the Bobcat and Alta trails.

Trail Notes

- Singletrack and fire trails
- Narrow and rocky in spots; short muddy sections on Rodeo Valley Trail in wet weather
- No dogs
- Bikes allowed on Coastal Fire Road
- Horses allowed on Rodeo Valley Trail and Coastal Fire Road
- No toilet or water at trailhead; toilet near Rodeo Lagoon, about 0.5-mile detour
- No fees

Head into picturesque Sausalito to fuel up at one of the many cafes and restaurants along the wharf.

The first thing you'll notice about the reddish, folded layers of rock at the Marin Headlands is that they almost match the color of the neighboring Golden Gate Bridge. Look more closely to discover the intricate layers, rows, and geometric shapes on these cliffs. The rocks you see are called chert, and they bear an intriguing history: chert is made up of billions of radiolarians—one-celled marine animals that form part of plankton. When they die, their skeletons accumulate on the ocean floor and form radiolarian ooze, which eventually hardens to become chert. The rich sepia-red color of the chert at the headlands distinguishes it from the grey and brown colors of most other chert, and is due to iron deposits in the ocean. Marin Headlands chert was actually formed thousands of miles to the south of where we see it today. As the Pacific Plate moved northward over millions of years, it was carried to its present location.

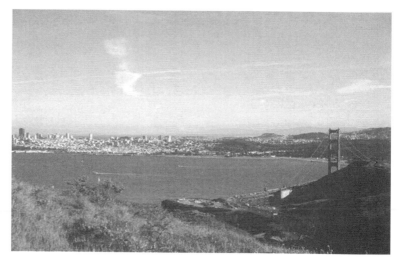

View of
San Francisco and
the bay from
SCA Trail at
Rodeo Valley

TENNESSEE VALLEY TRAILHEAD

On these two runs from the Tennessee Valley Trailhead you'll explore southeast/northwest-trending Coyote and Wolf ridges and the watercourses that separate them—Gerbode and Tennessee valleys and Green Gulch.

What You'll Find

The Tennessee Valley trailhead is no secret. The parking lot fills up early on weekday mornings, and on weekends, parked cars line the roadside. But don't be discouraged—once you're on the trail, you'll find relative peace and solitude. This trailhead's popularity isn't surprising—miles of trails extend north, south, and west, and provide numerous diverse loops.

You'll find toilets and a phone, but no water at the Tennessee Valley parking lot. The trailhead is usually well-stocked with GGNRA trail maps. (Note that distances are given in kilometers with miles in parentheses.) A large map posted on a park bulletin board tells you which trails allow bikes, horses, and/or dogs. (From Rodeo Lagoon, dogs are allowed on Lower Miwok Trail to Wolf Ridge, Wolf Ridge Trail, and Coastal Trail from Wolf Ridge to Rodeo Lagoon. From Tennessee Valley, dogs are allowed on Miwok Trail, north). You can also find this information and more at the GGNRA visitor center on Bunker Road in Rodeo Valley, open daily from 9:30 AM to 4:30 PM.

6

GERBODE VALLEY LOOP

The Marin Headlands' exposed ridges provide glorious views of the bay and coast on this route. Open grassy hillsides ripple toward the Pacific and dip to meet the coast at Tennessee Cove, where white breakers cap the stark blue ocean; a fog bank often hovers just off land. Smooth singletrack and fire trails traverse these coastal ridges and valleys on stiff climbs and gentle descents.

Distance	7.5 miles
Time	1-2 hours
Type	loop
High Point/Low Point	1001′/30′
Difficulty	moderate
Use	moderate
Maps	GGNRA maps at trailhead
Area Management	Golden Gate National Recreation Area

Trailhead Access From Hwy. 101, take the Stinson Beach/Hwy. 1 exit. Southbound travelers turn right immediately after exiting, and then left on Shoreline Hwy. at the stoplight. Northbound drivers cross beneath the freeway and continue straight at the stoplight. In less than 0.5 mile, turn left onto Tennessee Valley Rd. and follow it to the end.

At the western end of the parking lot, where the paved trail to Tennessee Valley Cove begins, there is a signpost with a map and pertinent information, as well as maps you can pick up to carry on the trail.

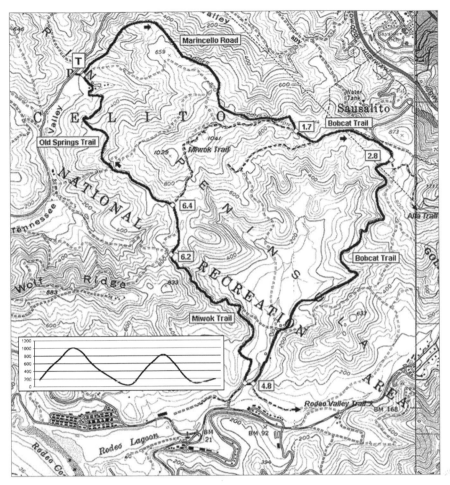

GERBODE VALLEY LOOP

Begin at east end of Tennessee Valley parking area. Turn left on dirt road to stables. Turn left on **Marincello Road.** (If you arrive at the stables, you've gone too far.)

Route Directions

1.7 Turn left on **Bobcat Trail.**

2.2 Pass trail to Hawk Backpack Camp.

2.8 Stay straight (right) on Bobcat at junction with Alta Trail.

4.8 Pass Rodeo Valley Trail. Turn right to cross bridge. Turn right again immediately on **Miwok Trail.**

6.2 Turn right at ridgetop to continue on Miwok Trail.

6.4 Turn left on **Old Springs Trail.**

About the Trail

Begin your climb out of Tennessee Valley on the wide, gravelly Marincello Road, what was to be the entrance road for the proposed Marincello community. Coyote bush borders the trail, and in spring, poppies, buttercup, and lupine add brilliant color in orange, yellow, and blue. Views improve with every step as you near the ridgetop: the municipalities of Marin, the hills of West Marin, Angel Island, Tiburon, the Richmond–San Rafael Bridge with the East Bay hills beyond, and even Mt. Diablo are visible on clear days.

At the ridge you join the Bobcat Trail, where you can stretch your legs on a slight downhill grade. Gerbode Valley spreads before you: serpentine rocks jut from the valley's low vegetation and a line of riparian willows runs through its middle. Beyond the valley is the Pacific, and to the south, the buildings of San Francisco. Look behind you for a view of the three peaks of Mt. Tam. In spring, pink checkerbloom and blue-eyed grass join coyote bush along the trail.

You continue on the Bobcat Trail, still a wide, smooth trail, to descend through Gerbode Valley. The distinct reddish path of your return route cuts into the hills on the valley's opposite side. Near the valley's head, the trail parallels a creek lined by willows, their leaves golden in fall. You pass the Rodeo Valley Trail just before crossing the creek on a bridge.

Now you begin the exposed climb out of Gerbode Valley on the Miwok Trail. The collage of muted vegetation and rock outcroppings in the valley below you, and the brilliant lupine, suncups, and poppies along the trail, may distract you from the steady grade. At the ridgetop, continue on the Miwok Trail for a short segment, but before the steep climb ahead, turn left on the Old Springs Trail. Watch your footing on rocky sections along this singletrack. Take in your last views of Tennessee Cove to the west and Mt. Tamalpais to the north as you descend into Tennessee Valley.

Alternate Routes

The many trails at the headlands provide options for routes of varying lengths. If you want to avoid the descent into Gerbode Valley and the climb out, you can still take in great views of the valley and the coast on a 3.5-mile loop. Turn right at the ridgetop from the Marincello Trail. A steep, knee-grinding descent takes you to the Old Springs Trail. Turn right and return to the trailhead.

- Singletrack and fire trails
- Relatively smooth trails except for a short rocky section on the Old Springs Trail
- Bikes allowed
- Horses allowed
- Dogs allowed only on the Miwok Trail from Rodeo Valley to Wolf Ridge
- Toilet at trailhead
- No water
- No fees

Try the Dipsea Café for delicious pancakes, creative omelets and tofu scrambles, 10 delicious smoothie choices, plus sandwiches, salads, and freshly squeezed juices. You'll find it just west of Tennessee Valley Road on Shoreline Highway.

Between September and December, up to 21 different species of raptors (birds of prey) circle over the headlands as they pause on their migratory journey south. Hawks, eagles, and falcons glide through the sky on air currents called thermals. Since thermals only form over land, the birds congregate here to catch an updraft that will propel them over the open waters of the Golden Gate; they pick up another thermal on the other side and continue on their journey. Hawk Hill, at the head of Gerbode Valley, is considered the prime spot for raptor watching.

7

GREEN GULCH LOOP

Exposed singletrack and fire trails crisscross the northern headlands on this diverse route. You'll survey dramatic coastal views, inhale the pungent smells of seaside vegetation, and run by fields of organic vegetables at Green Gulch Farm.

Distance	8.9 miles
Time	1.25–2.25 hours
Type	loop
High Point/Low Point	1016′/38′
Difficulty	moderate
Use	heavy
Maps	GGNRA maps at trailhead
Area Management	Golden Gate National Recreation Area

Trailhead Access See Green Gulch Loop (Run 6)

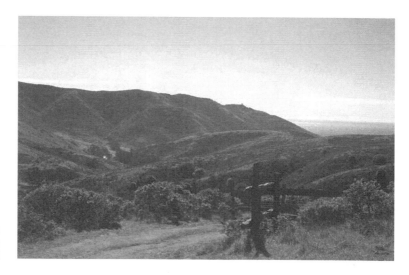

Looking towards the coast from the Miwok Trail

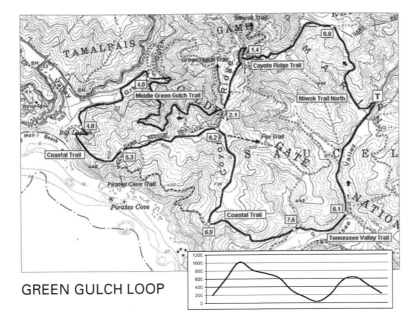

GREEN GULCH LOOP

Begin on the **Miwok Trail** at the northeast end of the parking lot. Follow Bay Area Ridge Trail signs to find it.

0.8 Junction. Stay straight/left on the Miwok Trail (spurs are shortcuts to the Coyote Ridge Trail).

1.4 Miwok Trail branches right. Leave Miwok and continue straight on unsigned **Coyote Ridge Trail.**

2.0 Pass Green Gulch Trail.

2.1 Turn right on **Middle Green Gulch Trail.**

4.0 Turn right through latched gate into Green Gulch Farm.

4.1 Turn left on dirt road at edge of field.

4.5 Go through gate at far west end of farm and turn left onto gravel road.

4.6 Turn right on unsigned **Coastal Trail.**

4.8 Turn left on Coastal Trail.

5.3 Go left on unsigned **Coyote Ridge Trail;** Coastal Trail (also called Pirates Cove Trail) branches right.

6.2 Turn right where **Coyote Ridge Trail** forks.

6.3 Continue straight/right where Fox Trail veers left.

6.9 Turn left on **Coastal Trail.**

7.6 Turn left on **Tennessee Valley Trail.**

8.1 Veer left on paved road.

About the Trail

Five trails link to create a loop that extends from Tennessee Valley to the coast and back. Begin on the Miwok Trail, a wide dirt singletrack that rises gently through low bushes of fragrant coyote bush, blackberry, grasses, and wild cucumber. Switchbacks temper the steepening incline as you climb toward the ridge. The trail levels and then descends briefly through a eucalyptus grove, before another short climb to the ridge.

Your route follows the Coyote Ridge Trail (unsigned) and the Miwok Trail branches right. You continue to climb on the ridgeline, although the steep spots are short. Sweet-smelling coastal scrub lines the trail and you have views northeast to Mt. Tamalpais and Blithedale Ridge, and east to Richardson Bay and Tiburon.

You descend into Green Gulch on a narrow and rutted singletrack. Large ceanothus bushes produce fragrant blue blossoms in spring, and sticky monkeyflower brightens the hillside. Watch your footing as you take in views of Muir Beach and Green Gulch Farm.

Green Gulch Farm occupies the fertile ravine below you. Primarily a Zen training temple, the center also operates a 7-acre vegetable farm and a 1-acre flower, herb, and fruit garden. At the edge of the farm, the trail becomes overgrown and is blocked by a gate. The accepted route to the Coastal Trail is through the farm. Enter the garden, pass the enticing fields of flowers and organic vegetables, and join the Coastal Trail at the far end of the farm.

Beyond Green Gulch, you head back up Coyote Ridge on the Coastal Trail, bypassing Muir Beach. (Continue the few hundred yards to the beach if you like, before turning left on the Coastal Trail.) The wide trail climbs steeply and unrelentingly along coastal bluffs, but each step provides more dramatic views of the inviting cove of Muir Beach. Waves crash against the cliffs below, and if you're lucky, fog drifts across the hillside, protecting you from the sun. Turkey vultures and hawks circle overhead in search of prey.

The singletrack Coastal Trail (or Pirates Cove Trail) branches right and heads south along the coastal bluffs. (Badly eroded in parts, with several steep ups and downs, this trail is not recommended for runners. Additionally, it is narrow and often crowded with hikers.) Your trail continues its steep ascent toward the ridgetop and then levels before one last grind. Look behind you for great views of the rugged coast along Pirate's Cove.

At the ridgetop, San Francisco's skyscrapers peek between a dip in the southern ridges of the headlands. You begin to descend toward the ocean; when you reach the coastal bluff, look over the edge to the rugged beach far below. On a clear day, you'll have views up and down the coast from this point.

As you descend the Coastal Trail into the wide girth of Tennessee Valley, look west for a dramatic view of the stark cliffs and dark sand of Tennessee Cove. Your red-earth trail is a little slippery at times, but is steep for only a short section and you can soon stretch your legs on an easy downhill. Look for quail scurrying off the trail. Lichen-covered rock outcroppings protrude from coastal scrub here. You meet the Tennessee Valley Trail and begin to parallel a willow-lined creek that runs through the valley. From here, your return to the trailhead is on a mostly level trail with only a slight incline.

Alternate Routes

You can easily shorten this route to a 4.7-mile loop by continuing on the Coyote Ridge Trail instead of turning right on the Middle Green Gulch Trail. Stay on Coyote Ridge toward the coast until you reach the Coastal Trail. Follow the featured route directions back to the trailhead.

Trail Notes

- Singletrack and fire trails
- Some narrow, rutted sections; Coastal Trail has a brief steep and possibly slippery downhill
- Dogs allowed on Miwok Trail North
- Bikes allowed on all trails on route; uphill only on Middle Green Gulch Trail
- Horses allowed on all trails on route
- Toilet at trailhead
- No water
- No fees

See Gerbode Valley Loop (Run 6) for details on the Dipsea Café.

History Notes

Tennessee Cove gets its name from the steamship *Tennessee,* which went aground here, having missed the Golden Gate on a foggy night in 1853.

MT. TAMALPAIS

From distant and disparate points around the bay, Mt. Tamalpais rises as an unmistakable landmark from the low coastal mountains that stretch north of the Golden Gate. Mt. Tam is a mecca for Bay Area outdoor enthusiasts: hikers, mountain bikers, and runners traverse the 200 miles of trails that cover the mountain. The mountain is the site of the notorious Dipsea Race—7.1-miles (with over 2000 feet of elevation gain and loss) from Mill Valley to Stinson Beach—an annual run since 1905.

Mt. Tam covers a 60-square-mile area, overlooking San Francisco, Marin, the East Bay, the Marin Headlands, the Pacific Ocean, and San Francisco and San Pablo bays. Three peaks compose its L-shaped ridge: At 2571 feet, East Peak is highest; West Peak stands 2567 feet, and Middle Peak is 2490 feet. Tamalpa Ridge extends west from West Peak to Bolinas Ridge, and three spur ridges extend from the mountain—Throckmorton to the south, Blithedale to the southeast, and Rocky Ridge to the north.

Wisps of fog often envelop the mountain's coastal trails; fragrant chaparral covers shiny serpentine expanses, and rare wildflowers bloom on forested slopes, making Mt. Tam seem many miles from any urban scene. Yet these 160 trails are in the middle of a megapolis. Only 10 miles from downtown San Francisco, and literally in the backyard of many Marin County residents, the mountain epitomizes an easily accessible natural area.

Although Mt. Tamalpais remains a prominent natural feature, humans have significantly altered the landscape, notably in the extensive network of well-maintained and well-signed trails that make Mt. Tam a runner's paradise. In the mid-1800s Lagunitas Creek was dammed to form Lake Lagunitas, the first of the five dammed watershed lakes in the area. Eldridge Grade, now a popular trail, was built in 1884 as the first stage route up the mountain, and in 1896 steam-powered trains began to chug from Mill Valley to near East Peak. The railroad track, known as the crookedest in the world, was destroyed by fire in the 1920s and the track was torn up in 1930.

The two inns on the mountain, West Point Inn and Mountain Home Inn, were built in 1904 and 1912, respectively. During the Depression, the Civilian Conservation Corps changed the landscape of the mountain with the construction of the Mountain Theater and many fire roads. Mt. Tam's peaks have also seen their share of construction. The fire lookout on East Peak was built as a marine obser-

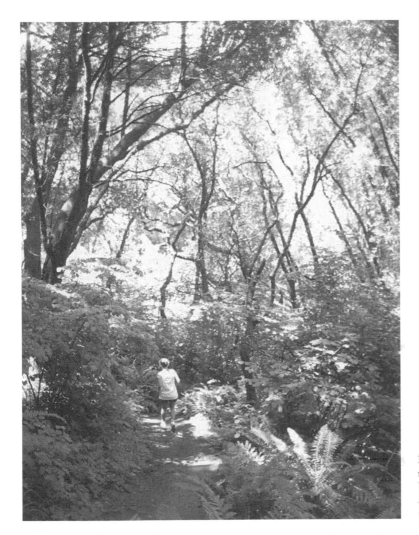

Runner on the
sun-dappled
Dipsea Trail in
Muir Woods
(Run 8)

vatory in 1901. West Peak once dominated the mountain's three
peaks at 2604 feet, but in 1951 the government bulldozed the summit to build the Mill Valley Air Force Station. The buildings have
since been torn down and the land now belongs to the Golden Gate
National Recreation Area.

Four managing agencies oversee Mt. Tamalpais. Trails in the
Marin Municipal Water District (MMWD), Mount Tamalpais State
Park, Muir Woods, and Marin Open Space District connect to form
an extensive network of routes with endless possibilities for runs of
all difficulties and distances. MMWD manages the most land: the Mt.

Tamalpais Watershed covers 18,500 acres—almost the entire north side of the mountain (plus across Bolinas-Fairfax Road to Pine Mountain and San Geronimo Ridge). Five reservoirs double as recreational lakes on the slopes of Mt. Tam: Phoenix, Alpine, Bon Tempe, Lagunitas, and Kent.

Mount Tamalpais State Park comprises the second largest amount of land—6400 acres—and encompasses most of the south side of the mountain (except Muir Woods). Muir Woods, although the smallest area of land on the mountain with only 560 acres, is the most-visited part of Mt. Tam. This majestic grove is the only remaining stand of old-growth redwoods in the Bay Area, where redwoods once grew in abundance. In the early 1900s, when development threatened land on Mt. Tamalpais, concerned residents recognized the importance of this forest. William Kent, already a large landowner on the mountain, bought the uncut redwoods in what would become Muir Woods, and later donated the land to the federal government. The Dipsea Trail skirts the heavily touristed center of Muir Woods.

Weather can vary dramatically on Mt. Tam, depending on which slope you're on and at what elevation. Choose a route according to the time of year and the weather conditions you desire. Summer fog often conceals the mountain's coastal slopes, although it usually lifts for a few mid-day hours. Fog frequently cools the southern slopes as well, near Muir Woods. Eastern slopes sometimes receive fog from the San Francisco Bay, but it generally burns off by late morning. You can count on the northern slopes to be virtually fog-free in summer.

Fall usually brings warm, clear days with far-reaching views up and down the coast. This can be the hottest time of year on the mountain, as in all of the Bay Area. Come winter, rain falls heaviest on the eastern slopes, turning the dry land a deep green. The valley fog that gathers in winter is more likely to envelop the mountain's eastern side than its coastal slopes. Warm spring days encourage bountiful wildflowers; many plants are in bloom by February. As temperatures warm, the hills gradually become a shimmering golden-brown, and by May, the summer fog pattern returns.

What You'll Find   **Mount Tamalpais State Park:** Trails in the state park are well marked, but remember that on signposts, the trail name is in small letters across the top and the destination is below, in larger letters. Toilets and water are located at most trailheads and at some locations along the trails. Check individual runs for specifics. No dogs are allowed on any of the trails in the state park. Bikes are permitted on fire roads, but not on singletrack trails. Horses are allowed on fire roads and some strategic connector trails.

State park trails are open daily from 7 AM to sunset: in winter, trails close as early as 6 PM and in summer, as late as 9 PM Park headquarters are at Pantoll Ranger Station.

Marin Municipal Water District: Toilets and water are available at various spots along MMWD trails. Check individual runs for specifics. Dogs are permitted on leash on all MMWD lands. Bikes are allowed on fire roads, but not on singletrack trails. Horses are allowed on many trails; check individual runs.

MMWD lands are open from sunrise to sunset. They may be closed under extremely hazardous fire conditions.

Muir Woods: The crowds at Muir Woods (and the paved trail through its center) make it less than ideal for running. Pass through the woods on the Dipsea Trail or connect to other trails, but otherwise, visit these impressive trees at a more leisurely pace. Toilets and facilities are available. Dogs, horses, and bikes are not allowed.

See the separate Marin Open Space District section for more information about MOSD trails on Mt. Tam.

8

MOUNTAIN HOME LOOP

This is Mt. Tam at its best: singletrack trails hug grassy hillsides with ocean views and pass through shaded redwood forests with moist creek ravines. You'll skirt legendary Muir Woods, traverse 3 miles of the notorious Dipsea Trail, and return via historic Mt. Tam trails.

Distance	9.9 miles
Time	1.25–2.5 hours
Type	loop
High Point/Low Point	1261´/131´
Difficulty	strenuous
Use	moderate
Maps	map $1 at Pantoll Ranger Station
Area Management	Mount Tamalpais State Park

Trailhead Access
From Hwy. 101, take the Shoreline Hwy. (Hwy. 1) exit. Turn left at the stoplight after about a mile, following signs to Mt. Tam and Stinson Beach. After 2.7 miles, veer right on Panoramic Hwy. At a fork after 0.8 mile, stay straight/gentle left on Panoramic Hwy. Continue to Mountain Home Inn. Park in the roadside lot across from the inn.

Route Directions
Walk south along Panoramic Hwy. a few hundred yards and begin running on the **Panoramic Trail** (Camp Eastwood Rd. joins the highway at the trailhead).

0.1 Pass Ocean View Trail.

0.4 Veer right on **Redwood Trail**.

1.0 Turn left at Tourist Club on a dirt road signed to SUN TRAIL. Turn right on **Sun Trail.**

1.8 Turn right sharply on **Dipsea Trail**, signed to MUIR WOODS.

2.0 Cross Muir Woods Rd. and pick up the Dipsea on the other side.

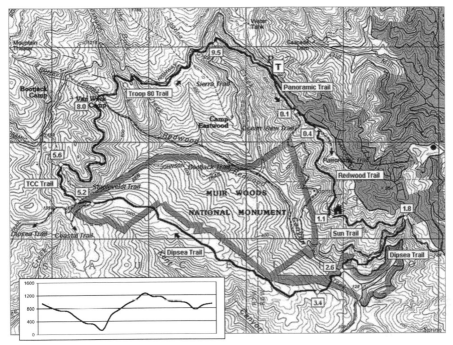

MOUNTAIN HOME LOOP

2.6 Cross Muir Woods Rd. again and run through Muir Woods parking lot. Follow signs to Dipsea Trail.
Turn right on the Dipsea, descend steps.

3.0 Cross double-plank bridge. Deer Park Fire Trail joins the Dipsea and the two run nearly parallel.

5.0 Veer left on Dipsea Trail where it diverges from Deer Park Fire Trail at sign marked DIPSEA TRAIL TO STINSON BEACH.
Turn right on **TCC Trail** (signed TCC TRAIL in small letters, TO STAPLEVELDT TRAIL in large letters).

5.6 Pass junction to Stapleveldt Trail and continue on TCC (SIGNED TO BOOTJACK).

8.0 Turn right at Van Wyck Meadow. Head left across the meadow on **Troop 80 Spur Trail.**

8.1 Continue straight on **Troop 80 Trail** at trail junction.

9.5 Turn left on Camp Eastwood Rd. and return to trailhead.

Your route begins on a narrow singletrack just below Panoramic
Hwy. Within the first mile you'll pass through shaded forests of redwood and bay laurel trees, and lope across open grassy hillsides with
stunning ocean views. In spring, brilliant blue-purple lupine, shiny
yellow buttercups, and bright orange Indian paintbrush lavish the
hillside. Poison oak thrives along this trail, and the shiny green or red
foliage or dry sticks (depending on the season) seek your bare arms
and legs. On a level grade or gentle descent the trail passes through
moist forests where creeks trickle down culverts and over grassy or
chaparral-covered slopes. In the spring, look for the bright yellow
blossoms of bush poppy, growing among chamise and coyote bush
on the hotter hillsides. Sweet smells drift by as you pass ceanothus
shrubs and oak trees.

Your route dips into a ravine and meets the Dipsea Trail. You
descend the first of many series of steps and continue downhill more
steeply to Muir Woods. The lush forest of redwood, oak, and bay laurel is alive with vibrant shades of green in springtime. Watch for poison oak growing along the sides of the trail!

Towering redwoods and moss-covered bay laurel shade the steep
half-mile climb out of Muir Woods, and ferns line the moist trail. You
meet the Deer Park Fire Road after exiting the woods, and for the
next mile and a half the Dipsea and Deer Park Fire Road run nearly
parallel to each other. If poison oak cramps your running on the singletrack Dipsea, opt for the wide fire trail. Rolling coastal hills covered with oak trees and coyote bush, views of the Marin Headlands,
spring wildflowers, and a strong ocean breeze propel you up the gentle incline along this section of the trail.

Beyond these open grasslands (called Hogsback for the curve of
their slope in profile), a redwood forest provides a cool break. You
complete your stint on the Dipsea with a stiff climb partway up the
infamous Cardiac Hill. You turn on the flat TCC (Tamalpais
Conservation Club) Trail before reaching Cardiac Hill's crest, but if
you haven't had enough uphill, continue to the top of the grade for
dramatic views of San Francisco and the Pacific.

The remaining 3 miles of this loop are on the mostly level TCC
and Troop 80 trails. They are smooth dirt singletracks, but watch for
occasional roots. The TCC crosses numerous wooden bridges over
small creeks (be careful of slippery wet wood) and winds in and out
of gulches. Tall redwoods provide shade for you and for lush ferns
and huckleberry. You pick up the Troop 80 Trail after the unlikely

grassy expanse of Van Wyck Meadow. The trail crosses dry slopes of manzanita, tanbark oak, and madrone and passes through moist redwood forests. Although you can't see it, you're running below and roughly parallel to Panoramic Highway.

The loop ends with a short section on paved Camp Eastwood Road that climbs back to Mountain Home.

Alternate Routes

For a shorter route (about 6 miles), and one that takes you into the heart of Muir Woods, turn right on the Ocean View Trail—the first trail you meet along the Panoramic Trail—and descend into the canyon on this shaded singletrack. Turn right on the main paved trail when you reach Muir Woods (you may have to dodge crowds) until you reach the singletrack Bootjack Trail. Follow it to Van Wyck Meadow and see the featured Route Directions to return to the trailhead.

Trail Notes

- Singletrack trails
- Narrow in spots; some root obstacles; wooden bridge crossings; poison oak
- No dogs
- No bikes
- Horses allowed on Deer Park Fire Road
- Toilet and water at trailhead, the Tourist Club, and Muir Woods
- No fees
- Popular trailhead and trails, especially through Muir Woods
- After heavy rains, water often floods the plank bridge over the creek in Muir Woods, and crossing is impossible. Call (415) 388-2596 to check the water level.

The Mountain Home Inn at the trailhead is your closest food source. A fixture on Mt. Tam since 1912, the inn serves food and drink on an outdoor deck that hosts terrific views toward the coast and the bay.

For a more casual atmosphere, head down the mountain to Mill Valley and check out Mama's Royal Café for a gut-filling meal. Fill up on Mama's omelets, pancakes, and French toast *after* a run.

You'll also find a few grocery stores in Mill Valley, including Whole Foods and Safeway on Miller Avenue, if you want something to go.

Nature Notes

A narrow, 450-mile strip of coast between central California and southern Oregon is the last remaining coast redwood habitat in the world. *Sequoia sempervirens*, or coast redwoods, thrive in the mild coastal climate, where heavy winter rains and cool summer fog provide ample moisture. Redwoods were once found throughout North America and on the coasts of Europe and Asia, but as the climates changed, their range became restricted to this fringe along the Pacific Ocean.

Coast redwoods are the tallest and the oldest trees in the world. Average height is 200 to 240 feet, and some reach 360 feet. Under favorable conditions, redwoods can live for more than 2,000 years. The tallest redwood measures 367.8 feet and grows in Redwood National Park, in northern California.

9

PANTOLL LOOP

This diverse and dramatic loop showcases some of the Bay Area's premier scenery, spectacular in every season and all weather conditions. An exposed singletrack path winds along steep coastal cliffs, a wide fire roads traverses shaded Douglas-fir forests, and a narrow trail crosses serpentine chaparral slopes on Mt. Tam's eastern flank.

Distance	7.7 miles
Time	1-2 hours
Type	loop
High Point/Low Point	2242'/1463'
Difficulty	moderate
Use	moderate
Maps	map $1 at Pantoll Ranger Station
Area Management	Mount Tamalpais State Park; Marin Municipal Water District

Trailhead Access

From Hwy. 101, take the Shoreline Hwy. (Hwy. 1) exit. Turn left at the stoplight after about a mile, following signs to Mt. Tam and Stinson Beach. After 2.7 miles, veer right on Panoramic Hwy. At a fork after 0.8 miles, stay straight/gentle left on Panoramic Hwy. Continue for another 4.6 miles to Pantoll Ranger Station. Turn left into the parking lot (parking fee). Or turn right on Pantoll Road at the Ranger Station to a small roadside parking area immediately on the right (no fee).

Cross Panoramic Highway to stairs that lead to the **Matt Davis Trail.**
Begin running on Matt Davis Trail.

1.4 Continue straight on Matt Davis Trail.

1.7 Continue straight on **Coastal Trail** (also the Bay Area Ridge Trail) as Matt Davis Trail branches left.

3.3 Turn right on **Willow Camp Fire Rd.**

3.4 Cross Ridgecrest Blvd.; begin running on **Laurel Dell Fire Rd.** on other side of metal gate.

4.0 Laurel Dell Meadow; continue straight on Laurel Dell Fire Rd. toward Potrero Meadow; Cataract Trail crosses fire road.

4.3 *Turn left on Old Stove Trail for a brief singletrack alternate.*

4.7 *Rejoin Laurel Dell Fire Rd. Turn left and continue toward Potrero Meadow.*

5.2 Turn right on **Benstein Trail.**

5.7 Turn right at junction with **Lagunitas Rd.**

5.8 Veer right on **Benstein Trail**, signed to ROCK SPRING.

6.0 Continue on Benstein Trail.

6.3 Veer left (still on Benstein Trail) to Rock Spring at junction with Simmons Trail.

6.4 Turn left at **Rock Spring** parking lot; run through lot; cross Ridgecrest Blvd. to join **Mountain Theater Fire Rd.** on other side of white metal gate.

6.5 Continue straight at junction with **Old Mine Trail**, signed to PANTOLL.

7.3 Turn right to continue on Old Mine Trail at junction with Riding and Hiking Trail.

7.7 Turn right on **Old Stage Rd.**, a few hundred feet from Pantoll trailhead.

About the Trail From Pantoll Ranger Station, the Matt Davis Trail (also called the Coastal Trail on the Olmstead map) winds over smooth dirt—only the occasional large root or rock impedes your gait. A canopy of Douglas-fir, oak, and bay laurel shades the first mile and you may see the treasured Calypso orchid in the sparse understory. The several rocky creekbeds that cross the trail flow with water in winter, but are no more than a trickle by late spring.

The trail leaves the shady forest cover and emerges on an open coastal hillside that drops steeply to the ocean. In spring, green slopes vibrate with colorful poppies, blue dicks, and lupine, joined by buttercups and blue-eyed grass. In summer and fall, the golden hillsides

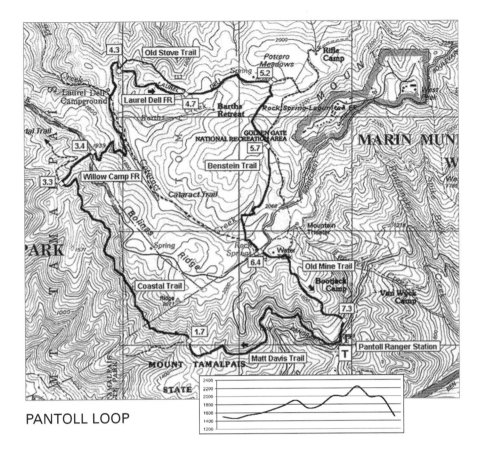

PANTOLL LOOP

contrast with deep green foliage of bay laurel and oak that pocket the slopes. The trail winds in and out of shaded gullies, crowded by thick stands of trees. Narrow in spots, the path requires careful attention to footing. On clear days, you'll have views of the entire Bay Area, from Pacifica to Point Reyes and Mt. Diablo to the Farallones. The familiar coastal fog often rides ocean breezes and sweeps up the mountain's slopes, creating a magical environment.

The Matt Davis Trail branches left, headed for the coast; you continue on the Coastal Trail and find yourself high above Stinson Beach, where white-capped waves crash on a wide sandy expanse. Your view now extends north, beyond smooth grassy hills and rocky outcroppings, to Bolinas Lagoon and Inverness Ridge.

Bid farewell to your coastal views when you turn on Willow Camp Fire Road. A short climb takes you to the Laurel Dell Fire Road, across Ridgecrest Blvd. Now on Marin Municipal Water

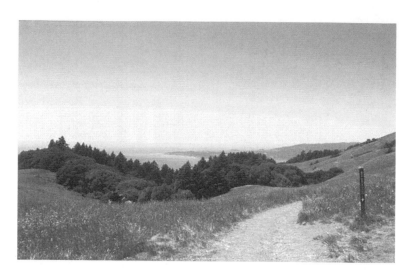

Coast Trail,
Mt. Tamalpais

District land, you begin to wind your way to the east side of Mt. Tam. The smooth Laurel Dell Fire Road descends and then levels in a Douglas-fir forest. It crosses a creek (you may have to rock-hop) in the clearing and picnic area of the same name, and continues to Potrero Meadow.

If you tire of wide fire roads, take a brief detour on the Old Stove Trail, which rejoins the Laurel Dell Fire Road after a short distance. This fun diversion begins steeply and becomes a narrow trail through dense chaparral over serpentine rock. Tall manzanita and ceanothus crowd the trail, and sticky monkeyflower, Indian paintbrush, and soaproot line the edges.

The Laurel Dell Fire Road crosses this same landscape; the green/grey swath of trail and reddish decomposing soil signal the presence of serpentine rock. Your view here sweeps across the hills of northern and eastern Marin to Mt. Diablo in the East Bay, taking in the bay and the Richmond-San Rafael Bridge.

From Potrero Picnic Area, the Benstein Trail climbs through a thick Douglas-fir forest to a serpentine outcropping, where manzanita and dwarf Sargent cypress trees are among the few plants that survive the inhospitable serpentine soil. Pay careful attention to your footing through this rocky and root-strewn stretch. The trail then descends gently through a peaceful light forest, shaded by oak, bay laurel, and madrone. The impressive patch of greenish serpentine (called Serpentine Swale) in the meadow below you comes into view as you approach Rock Spring.

Across the Rock Spring parking area (now back in Mount Tamalpais State Park), you descend an open hillside to return to the trailhead. Lupine and buttercups paint the hillside in spring, among fragrant stands of bay laurel and oaks. Views are outstanding: San Francisco and the Marin Headlands; the East Bay to Mt. Diablo; Tiburon and Belvedere; and the southeastern flank of Mt. Tam, where Old Railroad Grade winds up the mountain.

For a shorter route (6.5 miles), turn right on the Cataract Trail from Laurel Dell picnic area. The shaded trail follows Cataract Creek for 1.2 miles to reach Rock Spring. From there, follow the featured run's return route to the trailhead.

Alternate Routes

Another option is a short out-and-back along the Coastal Trail— a rewarding run in itself, especially when spring wildflowers are in full bloom.

Trail Notes

- Singletrack and fire trails
- Narrow trails; some rocks and roots, especially on Benstein Trail; muddy in isolated patches after wet weather, but not sticky
- No bikes
- Horses allowed on Laurel Dell Fire Road and Old Mine Trail
- No dogs in Mount Tamalpais State Park; dogs on leash in MMWD
- Restrooms and water at Pantoll Ranger Station; toilet at Laurel Dell; toilet at Potrero Camp; toilet at Rock Spring
- Parking fee in Pantoll lot; no fee at pull-out with limited parking across from Pantoll on Ridgecrest Blvd.
- On warm weekends, be prepared for a lot of company on these trails. The earlier you start, the fewer people you'll have to pass, and the fewer parking hassles you'll encounter.

See Mountain Home Loop (Run 8) for food suggestions.

Nature Notes

The line of white sand along Stinson Beach has an interesting story behind it: Whereas beach sand is usually composed of sediment from the rocks on the cliffs bordering the beach, the stark Stinson sand strip comes from the granitic rocks at Point Reyes, a few miles to the north. The sediment is carried by currents that flow south from Point Reyes, sweep around Bolinas Point, and deposit the granitic granules on the beach.

The delicate Calypso orchid (*Calypso bulbosa*) grows in shady areas along the Matt Davis, Laurel Dell, and Benstein trails. You may see no more than a glimpse of lavender in the forest understory as you run past.

See **Nature Notes** for the Northside Loop (Run 12) to find out about the serpentine rocks along the Laurel Dell Fire Road and the Benstein Trail.

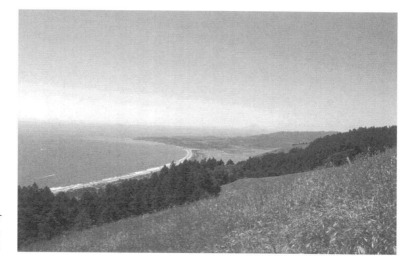

View of
Stinson Beach
from Coastal Trail

10

PHOENIX LAKE LOOP

Phoenix Lake lies at the base of the northern slopes of Mt. Tam and is an ideal starting point for exploring the mountain's lower flanks. You'll have impressive views of the peaks; climb steep, exposed slopes; descend through oak woodlands and moist redwood forests; and enjoy spring wildflowers. Although this is a busy trailhead and the main fire grades are heavily used, the singletrack trails provide a surprising feeling of "wildness" for such an accessible area.

Distance	5.8 miles
Time	0.75–1.5 hours
Type	loop
High Point/Low Point	679'/107'
Difficulty	moderate
Use	heavy
Maps	MMWD Mt. Tamalpais Watershed Map at Sky Oaks Ranger Station
Area Management	Marin Municipal Water District

Trailhead Access

Entry to the Phoenix Lake trailhead is through Natalie C. Greene Park in the city of Ross. From Hwy. 101, take Sir Francis Drake Blvd. 2.5 miles to Lagunitas Rd. (at the Marin Art & Garden Center). Lagunitas Rd. ends at the Natalie C. Greene Park parking lot.

NOTE: Parking is often difficult at this popular trailhead, especially on weekends. Do not park in undesignated spots or anywhere near a "no parking" sign. The lot is patrolled and cars are ticketed throughout the day. If the lot is full, you'll have to park some distance down Lagunitas Road and walk or run—a dirt path parallels the road—to the trailhead.

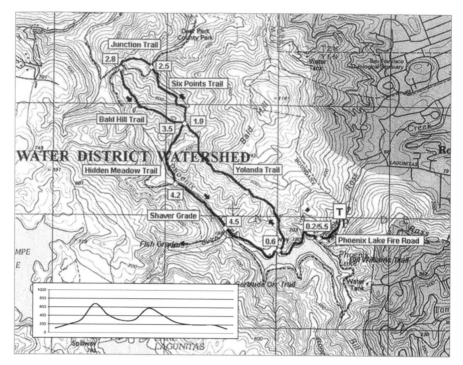

PHOENIX LAKE LOOP

Route Directions

Begin on the fire road from the parking lot.

0.2 Continue straight (northwest) on **Phoenix Lake Fire Rd.**, signed to LAKE LAGUNITAS.

0.3 Pass Worn Springs Rd.

0.6 Turn right on **Yolanda Trail.**

1.9 Six Points junction; take the second trail from right, the unsigned **Six Points Trail.**

2.5 Continue straight across Deer Park Fire Rd. to **Junction Trail.**

2.8 Boy Scout junction; go straight on singletrack (unsigned) **Bald Hill Trail** across Deer Park Fire Rd. (Canyon, Moore, and Ridge trails also converge here).

3.5 Six Points junction; turn right sharply on **Hidden Meadow Trail.**

4.2 Turn left on **Shaver Grade.**

4.5 Continue straight on **Phoenix Lake Fire Rd.**

5.5 Turn left at dam and retrace your steps to trailhead.

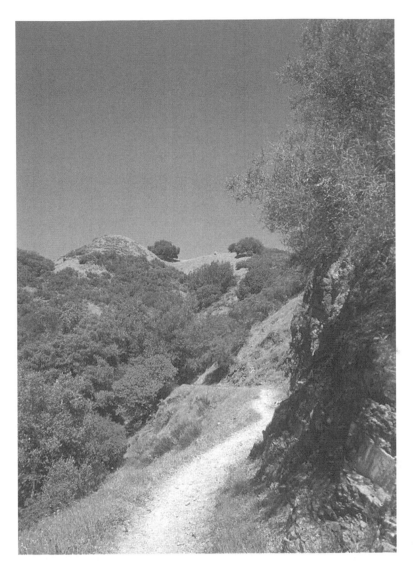

Yolanda Trail

A wide fire road leads to the Phoenix Lake Dam from Natalie C. Greene Park. The road crests at the dam, where an interpretive sign includes a map of the area. Stay right on the Phoenix Lake Fire Road; after about half a mile, turn on the Yolanda Trail to escape the bikers and hikers that frequent the fire road. You climb through a sparse forest of oak, bay laurel, and madrone on this exceptional singletrack. The trail is narrow, but its surface is well worn and provides good footing. In the spring, long tassels hang from the newly bud-

About the Trail

ding oaks, and brilliant wildflowers grow among native grasses. Milkmaids appear as early as January, and as the days grow longer and warmer, blue dicks, hound's tongue, California buttercups, Indian paintbrush, lupine, and poppies produce a colorful show.

The trail levels and leaves the cover of oak and bay laurel; exposed, grassy slopes drop steeply to your left. Look back for a view of the majestic peaks of Mt. Tam. As you spring along this trail, you'll feel far removed from the city just a few miles away.

The Yolanda Trail crests at Six Points Junction, and you descend gently on the soft-dirt Six Points Trail through a forest of bay laurel and redwood. Several small streambeds lined with moist ferns cross the trail. Across Deer Park Fire Road, you climb gently up an open, chaparral-covered slope on the Junction Trail. You may have to take large steps to hoist yourself over protruding rocks and roots. (During the rainy season, the Junction Trail may be a muddy river. Detour left on Deer Park Fire Road from the Six Points Trail, and continue to Boy Scout Junction.) The Junction Trail meets Deer Park Fire Road again at Boy Scout Junction, where you begin a stiff climb on the root-strewn Bald Hill Trail. Majestic oaks border the trail, and in early spring, baby blue eyes and shooting stars grow among bunchgrasses. When you reach the ridge, look for the smooth red bark of an unusually large madrone on your left.

You loop back to Six Points Junction on the Bald Hill Trail and descend a steep, grassy hillside on the narrow Hidden Meadow Trail. Sneak peeks at Mt. Tam as you wind down to the serene "hidden" meadow. As you enter an oak woodland, switchbacks ease the descent. You then cross a stream via a wooden bridge and enter a redwood flat where you join Shaver Grade. This wide, shaded trail shortly meets Phoenix Lake Fire Road. Pass Fish and Eldridge grades, which lead to Lake Lagunitas and the vast network of Mt. Tam trails, and return to the shores of Phoenix Lake.

Alternate Routes This trailhead provides plenty of alternate routes of varying length and difficulty—a short, level lakeside loop or longer, hilly routes that climb the flanks of Mt. Tam. For a short loop (about 2.7 miles) around Phoenix Lake on both singletrack and fire trails, combine the Tucker and Gertrude Ord trails (the Gertrude Ord Trail is called the Phoenix Lake Trail on some maps) and the Phoenix Lake Fire Road. Cross the dam at the head of the lake and follow the **Tucker Trail** (it turns into the Bill Williams Trail) for 0.5 mile, to the right-branching

Gertrude Ord Trail. A series of steps launches this singletrack trail, a relatively flat route with gentle ups and downs. A forest of oak, bay laurel, and madrone shades the trail, and the reservoir sparkles below. Shortly before meeting the **Phoenix Lake Fire Road,** you enter a dense redwood forest. Turn right at the next junction and follow this wide trail back to the dam.

If you want a longer run, head up Fish Grade to Lake Lagunitas and Bon Tempe Lake, or take Eldridge Grade toward East Peak. A simple way to extend the featured route is to add the loop around the lake: As you return to Phoenix Lake along Shaver Grade, turn right on the **Gertrude Ord Trail,** just past the multi-trail junction with Fish and Eldridge grades. Only a small sign indicating that no dogs or bikes are allowed marks the start of the trail. Turn left where Gertrude Ord meets the wide **Bill Williams Trail** and run 0.5 mile back to the fire road leading to the parking lot.

- Singletrack and fire road
- Some narrow trails; rock and root obstacles on Bald Hill, Six Points, and Junction trails; Junction Trail may be very muddy in rainy season—detour on Deer Park Fire Road
- Dogs on leash
- Bikes allowed on fire trails
- Horses allowed on all trails on this route
- Toilet at Natalie C. Greene Park
- No fees
- On weekends, Phoenix Lake is a popular hiking, biking, and running spot. Singletrack trails are less traveled than the fire roads.

Detour through the quaint town of Ross for a bite to eat at Café Marmalade. The small café serves espresso, baked goods, granola, and soups and sandwiches. To grab something on the go, try the Ross Grocery, a small but well-stocked corner store, with fresh fruit, juices, snacks, yogurt, cookies, and even deli sandwiches.

To get to both from Lagunitas Road, turn south onto Ross Commons. The corner store is one block ahead on the left, and the café is just a few doors beyond. No meters and 1 hour parking anytime—a rarity in the Bay Area!

11

ALPINE LAKE TRAVERSE

Follow singletrack trails along the shore of forested Alpine Lake and climb the slopes of Mt. Tam on gently rolling ups and downs through mixed forest. Complete this loop on an exposed fire trail across a serpentinite-riddled ridgetop.

Distance	6.4 miles
Time	0.75–1.5 hours
Type	loop
High Point/Low Point	1254′/672′
Difficulty	moderate
Use	light
Maps	MMWD Mt. Tamalpais Watershed Map (available at Sky Oaks Ranger Station)
Area Management	Marin Municipal Water District

Trailhead Access From Hwy. 101, take Sir Francis Drake Blvd. 5.3 miles to Pacheco Dr. in Fairfax and turn left (west). Turn right on Broadway and then left onto Bolinas Rd. Follow Bolinas Rd. for 1.5 miles to a difficult-to-spot turnoff on the left, signed to Bon Tempe Lake and Lake Lagunitas.

Continue to the entrance kiosk. Pay attendant or put fee in provided envelope. Continue to a gravel road signed to ALPINE AND BON TEMPE LAKES. Turn right and follow road to the first left turn, into a gravel parking lot.

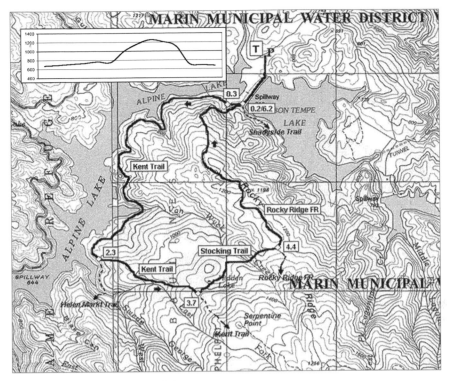

ALPINE LAKE TRAVERSE

From parking area, follow right-branching gravel road signed to Bon Tempe Dam Shady Side Trail. Cross dam.

0.2 Veer right on **Alpine-Bon Tempe Pump Fire Rd.** toward Kent Trail and Rocky Ridge Fire Rd.

0.3 Pass left-branching Rocky Ridge Fire Rd.

0.8 Veer left on **Kent Trail,** where Alpine-Bon Tempe Pump Fire Rd. dead-ends.

2.3 Turn left to continue on Kent Trail, signed to Potrero Meadow (Helen Markt Trail continues straight around Alpine Lake).

3.7 Turn left on **Stocking Trail.**

4.4 Turn left on **Rocky Ridge Fire Rd.**

6.2 At dam, continue straight across to return to trailhead.

About the Trail Mt. Tam looms above Bon Tempe Lake as you cross the dam to begin this route. On the far side of the dam, you pick up the wide, gravel Alpine-Bon Tempe Pump Fire Road and follow it to the southern tip of Alpine Lake. Here, you begin the singletrack Kent Trail along the lakeshore. Madrone, oak, and Douglas-fir initially offer shade, and their roots are frequent intruders on the otherwise smooth dirt trail.

You cross several rocky creekbeds and soon leave the trees on a gentle climb. The trail becomes rocky as it heads into chaparral, dominated by chamise and manzanita. Keep one eye on your footing and the other on great views of the densely forested slopes across Alpine Lake. Blue-eyed grass, buttercup, and false lupine bloom in spring.

You proceed along the lakeshore, winding in and out of finger-like inlets. Bunchgrasses, tanbark oak, huckleberry, and abundant spring iris thrive beneath the shady cover of oak, Douglas-fir, and madrone. Erosion threatens the narrow trail—in some spots the path slides precariously toward the lake. Chose your footing carefully to minimize impact.

The Kent Trail leaves Alpine Lake via a series of railroad-tie steps and climbs through a shady forest. It reaches drier terrain, where dense huckleberry bushes crowd the trail. Manzanita, tanbark oak, and tall madrone also grow here. The narrow trail arrives at a deep creek ravine, graced by tall slender redwoods. A steep, eroded hillside of red earth drops into the ravine on its far side. The sound of rushing water accompanies your steps until you leave the creekbed and climb into a thick forest.

You turn on the duff-covered Stocking Trail and continue beneath madrone, Douglas-fir, and redwood trees. The trail passes small, marshy Hidden Lake, where you might hear a chorus of frogs. As you approach Rocky Ridge, the trail and vegetation change. On a dark red, rocky path, you climb through dense chaparral composed of ceanothus, manzanita, sticky monkeyflower, and chamise to reach the Rocky Ridge Fire Road.

True to its name, the rocky fire road winds through a barren landscape of greenish serpentine bordered by low chaparral shrubs. In spring, white and blue ceanothus blossoms emit a sweet fragrance. The exposed trail allows extensive views—the three peaks of Mt. Tam rise behind you, Pine Mountain Ridge lies to your left, and the grassy knolls and forested gullies of Bolinas Ridge stave off coastal

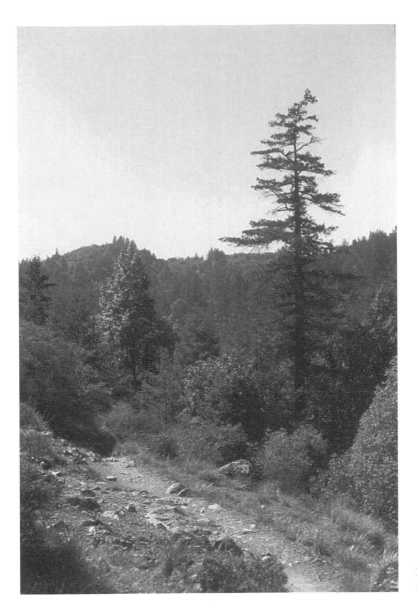

Kent Trail around
Alpine Lake

fog. Views of the bay extend south and all the way to the Delta in the east.

Small loose rocks on a steep downhill grade can make the trail slippery as you near Bon Tempe Lake. You descend into a lightly shaded forest and re-cross the dam to reach the trailhead.

Alternate Routes   To extend this run, explore the Helen Markt Trail, which follows the shore of Alpine Lake past the Kent Trail turnoff. Helen Markt ends at the Cataract Trail, which you can follow up the lush ravine of Cataract Creek. To loop back to the trailhead, take the High Marsh Trail to the Willow Trail to the Kent Trail, and follow the featured route back via the Stocking Trail and Rocky Ridge Fire Road.

Trail Notes
- Singletrack and fire trails
- Root and rock obstacles on the Kent Trail; steep and slippery downhill on Rocky Ridge Fire Road
- Dogs on leash
- Bikes allowed on Rocky Ridge Fire Road
- Horses allowed on Alpine-Bon Tempe Pump and Rocky Ridge fire roads
- Toilet at trailhead and far side of Bon Tempe Dam
- No water
- $5 parking fee
- No swimming—this is drinking water for Marin, so don't plan on a dip after a hot run

 Fairfax provides plenty of options for snacks or meals, before or after a run. The Fairfax Coffee Roasting Company, on the corner of Broadway and Bolinas, serves espresso drinks, Double Rainbow ice cream, croissants, and pastries, plus bagels, yogurt and granola, and sandwiches. Check out the Good Earth Natural Foods grocery across Sir Francis Drake Blvd. for organic fruits and vegetables, great bread and scones, bins with delicious munchies, and more.

12

NORTHSIDE LOOP

This challenging tour of the eastern flank of Mt. Tam will transport
you from serpentine moonscapes to coastal redwood forests, with
stunning views of the Bay Area throughout. The terrain is rocky and
requires careful attention to footing—recommended only if you
enjoy and are comfortable with technically challenging trails.

Distance	11.7 miles
Time	1.5–3 hours
Type	loop
High Point/Low Point	2040′/679′
Difficulty	strenuous
Use	light
Maps	MMWD Mt. Tamalpais Watershed Map
	at Sky Oaks Ranger Station
Area Management	Marin Municipal Water District

Trailhead Access

From Hwy. 101, take Sir Francis Drake Blvd. 5.3 miles to Pacheco
Dr. in Fairfax and turn left (west). Turn right on Broadway and then
left onto Bolinas Rd. Follow Bolinas Rd. for 1.5 miles to a difficult-
to-spot turnoff on the left, signed to Bon Tempe Lake and Lake
Lagunitas.

Continue to the entrance kiosk. Pay attendant or put fee in provided envelope. Continue to a gravel road signed to ALPINE AND
BON TEMPE LAKES. Turn right and follow it to the first left turn,
into a gravel parking lot.

From parking area, follow right-branching gravel road signed to BON TEMPE DAM SHADY SIDE TRAIL. Cross dam.

0.2 Veer right on **Alpine-Bon Tempe Pump Fire Rd.** toward Kent Trail and Rocky Ridge Fire Rd.

0.3 Go left on **Rocky Ridge Fire Rd**, signed to POTRERO MEADOW.

2.1 Turn right sharply on **Rock Spring Fire Rd.**, also signed to POTRERO MEADOW. Pass junctions for Upper Berry Trail, Lower Northside Trail, and Lagoon Fire Trail.

3.3 Rifle Camp; turn left on **Northside Trail.**

4.4 Continue straight on Northside Trail, signed for ELDRIDGE GRADE.

6.0 Inspiration Point; continue straight on **Eldridge Grade.**

6.7 Pass Wheeler Trail.

7.3 Pass Indian Fire Rd.

8.4 Turn left on **Lakeview Fire Rd.**; Eldridge Grade goes right to PHOENIX LAKE.

8.6 *Optional detour: Turn right on **Pilot Knob Trail**, then right again on **Lakeview Fire Rd.** from **Pilot Knob Trail.***

9.6 Turn right at Lake Lagunitas parking lot and run up paved road.

10.0 Turn right on **Pumpkin Ridge Trail** (where road curves to left).

10.4 Turn left on unsigned **Sky Oaks Trail.**

10.6 Cross road on spur trail to unsigned **Sunnyside Trail** and follow shoreline for 1.1 miles back to the trailhead.

About the Trail

From the trailhead at only 716 feet, Mt. Tam looks distant and unattainable, but you will shortly reach Inspiration Point at 2040 feet—this run's highest spot.

Across Bon Tempe Dam, you immediately begin to climb on a wide trail through madrone, oak, and Douglas-fir. In winter and early spring, the bare branches of deciduous oaks reveal wispy beards of moss; their light green color contrasts with the deep green firs in this mixed forest. You have views of the lake and of the grassy, rounded knobs of the Marin hills, interrupted by rocky outcroppings.

After a moderate climb, you reach one of this run's most dazzling features: a high expanse of glistening serpentine rock, characteristic of Mt. Tamalpais. Greenish rocks and dark red soil (serpentine turns red when it erodes) define the trail as it snakes into the distance

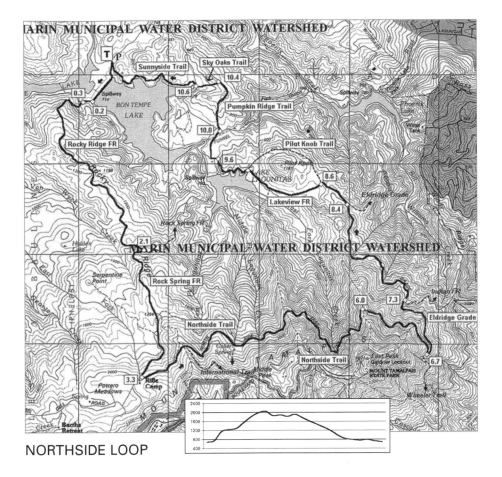

NORTHSIDE LOOP

toward majestic East Peak. Rocks litter the trail and low shrubs of red-barked manzanita and tufts of bunchgrasses surround serpentine rock outcroppings. In spring, purple and white ceanothus blossoms send sweet smells into the air.

The trail alternates between shaded and sunny stretches. Tanbark oak and toyon grow beneath Douglas-fir, and a thick fir scent rises from the earth. Several creeks pass under the trail. After a long, steady climb you reach Rifle Camp, the site of picnic tables, grills, and a toilet.

The Northside Trail, a level singletrack along the eastern flank of Mt. Tam, begins from Rifle Camp in a forest where oak, bay, and madrone strain to reach sunlight through towering Douglas-firs. Several creeks bubble across the trail in wet winters and springs, but are barely a trickle in summer and fall. You leave the trees to cross an open expanse of shiny serpentinite outcroppings and low manzanita. Gnarled dwarf cypress trees grow in the nutrient-poor serpentine soil, unchallenged by competitors.

The trail becomes extremely rocky and may be wet in the rainy season, making it slippery and somewhat treacherous. Sneak peeks at wide vistas of the Bay Area, from Marin to the East Bay, but don't let your eyes stray for long from the difficult footing.

Redwood trees soon replace serpentine rocks and vegetation, and are in turn replaced by an oak and madrone forest, where sunlight filters through the leaves.

You meet Eldridge Grade, at first a rocky trail in open chaparral, and head down the mountain; as you descend, you pass through moist redwood stands where ferns and evergreen huckleberry flank the wide span. Superb views of the bay nearly stop you in your tracks—from the San Rafael Bridge across Tiburon and Mill Valley to Mountain Home Inn on the southwestern slope of Mt. Tam.

You soon join Lakeview Fire Road. For a change of pace, take the singletrack Pilot Knob Trail over rolling hills studded with oaks and madrone. Fields of purple hound's tongue grace the beginning of the trail in spring. After a short climb through a shady oak and madrone forest, the duff-covered trail drops down to rejoin Lakeview Fire Road.

A short jaunt through the Lake Lagunitas parking lot and up the access road brings you to the Pumpkin Ridge Trail. Pause for a moment to look back at the impressive mountain whose slopes you have just crossed. Finish off this route on the shoreline Sunnyside Trail along Bon Tempe Lake, a narrow path between the lake and rolling grassy slopes.

Alternate Routes If you're looking for a shorter route, the Sky Oaks trailhead offers numerous options, including scenic and simple loops around Bon Tempe Lake and Lake Lagunitas.

Trail Notes
- Fire trail and singletrack
- Very rocky trails, especially parts of the Northside Trail, Rocky Ridge Fire Road, and Eldridge Grade
- Dogs on leash
- Bikes allowed on Rocky Ridge, Rock Spring, and Lakeview fire roads, and Eldridge Grade

- Horses allowed on all trails on this route, except the Pilot Knob Trail
- Toilets at trailhead, far side of Bon Tempe Dam, Rifle Camp, Lake Lagunitas parking lot
- Water at Lake Lagunitas parking lot
- $5 parking fee

See Alpine Lake Loop (Run 11) for Fairfax food suggestions.

Nature Notes

The expanses of greenish-grey rock you see on the Rocky Ridge Fire Road and the Northside Trail are serpentinite, the California state rock. Serpentinite is one of the distinctive geological formations that ripple the Bay Area landscape. As wind and rain weather the shiny rock, it decomposes into a brick-red soil. This soil's low nutrient content and high toxic-metal content make it inhospitable to most plants; those that survive have evolved tolerance mechanisms that allow them to grow and reproduce in the harsh serpentine environment. Thus, serpentine soils are often refuges for endemic and rare plants. Sargent cypress trees and Hooker's manzanita are two of the rare species found in serpentine soils on Mt. Tam.

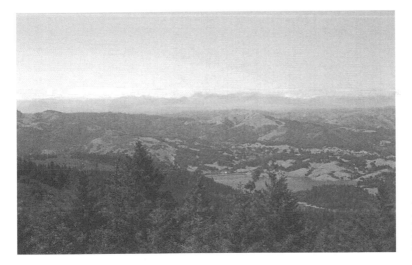

View of
Bon Tempe Lake
from the
Northside Trail

13

KENT LAKE OUT-AND-BACK

Are you looking for exceptional scenery and solitude without the ups and downs and obstacles on other Mt. Tam trails? Here's an out-and-back route above Kent Lake on a mostly level, smooth, and lightly used service road.

Distance	up to 9.6 miles
Time	up to 2.5 hours
Type	out-and-back
High Point/Low Point	645'/364'
Difficulty	easy to moderate
Use	light
Maps	MMWD Mt. Tamalpais Watershed Map at Sky Oaks Ranger Station
Area Management	Marin Municipal Water District

Trailhead Access From Hwy. 101, take Sir Francis Drake Blvd. 5.3 miles to Pacheco Drive in Fairfax and turn left (west). Turn right on Broadway and then left onto Bolinas Rd. Continue 7.5 miles to Alpine Dam. Park on the side of the road, just before crossing the dam. Do not block access to the service road.

Route Directions Begin on east side of Alpine Dam.
0.1 Continue straight where service road goes left.
2.0 Pass Old Vee Rd.
3.5 Pass two unsigned right-branching trails.
4.8 End of trail; retrace steps or see **Alternate Routes.**

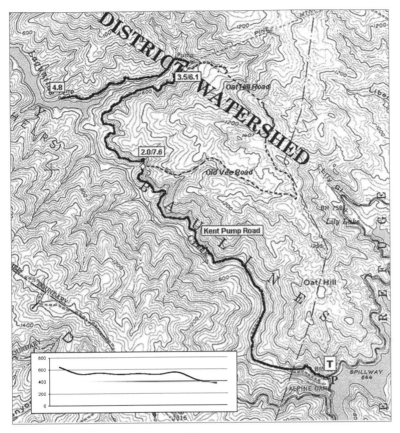

KENT LAKE OUT-AND-BACK

About the Trail

Alpine Lake Dam is only 7 miles west of Fairfax, but the area around it feels wild and remote. The imposing dam drops into a deep canyon with forested slopes rising high on both sides. Kent Pump Road begins just east of the dam, and continues above the ravine to the far southern finger of Kent Lake.

The trail begins on a short descent, but quickly levels and remains generally flat the entire route. Oak, madrone, and bay laurel shade the broad trail; big-leaf maple and tall redwoods soon join the forest, and their dense cover keeps the route remarkably cool. The trail becomes more exposed as it progresses, bordered by coyote bush, sticky monkeyflower, morning glory, and ceanothus. You pass a red-rock hillside covered with small, basal clusters of dudleya.

Several creekbeds descend the eastern hillside in small ravines and pass through culverts under the trail. Beyond the turnoff to Old Vee Road, you may catch a glimpse through the thinning forest of Kent Lake, far below. The trail curves northeast, tracing a finger of the lake, and enters more shade. You pass a small concrete building on the side of the trail and two unsigned trails branch right; a small sign indicates that your trail dead-ends in 0.5 mile. The trail ends at Kent Lake, where partially submerged dead trees create an eerie bleakness that contrasts with the thriving forest on the opposite hillside.

Alternate Routes Although one attraction of this out-and-back route is its simplicity, you can make it into a loop for a more challenging run. After 3.5 miles on the service road, two trails branch to the right. Turn on the first trail; after a quarter mile turn right again and begin a stiff climb—about 700 feet in about half a mile. Turn right on Oat Hill Road and continue to the junction with Old Vee Road. Descend steeply on Old Vee Road to Kent Pump Road and retrace your steps to Alpine Dam.

Trail Notes
- Unpaved service road
- Smooth trail
- Dogs allowed
- Bikes allowed
- Horses allowed
- No facilities
- No fees
- Great for jogging strollers

   See Alpine Lake Loop (Run 11) for food suggestions in Fairfax.

14

BOLINAS RIDGE

The Bolinas Ridge Trail begins just north of Mt. Tamalpais, sneaks through towering redwoods, breaks into open chaparral, and sweeps over rolling grasslands to reach Sir Francis Drake Boulevard in West Marin. Views of Bolinas Lagoon, Tomales Bay, and the Pacific Ocean are highlights of this trail. Two trailheads provide multiple options: an 11-mile shuttle run, shorter out-and-back runs from either entry point, or a near-marathon length out-and-back. You may be in full sun on Bolinas Ridge, while the coast, just a few miles away, is soaked in dense fog.

Distance	11.1 miles one way; up to 22.2 miles
Time	up to 5.5 hours
Type	shuttle or out-and-back
High Point/Low Point	1662′ /358′
Difficulty	easy to strenuous
Use	light
Maps	Point Reyes National Seashore South District trail map at visitor center (partial route shown)
Area Management	Golden Gate National Recreation Area (Bolinas Ridge is part of the GGNRA but is managed by Point Reyes National Seashore—contact Point Reyes visitor center for information about the trail)

Trailhead Access

Southern Trailhead: From Hwy. 101, take Sir Francis Drake Blvd. 5.3 miles to Pacheco Dr. in Fairfax and turn left (west). Turn right on Broadway and then left onto Bolinas Rd. Continue past Alpine Dam (at about 7.5 miles) to Ridgecrest Blvd. (9.0 miles). Park on the side of the road. The trail begins just north of the junction.

Northern Trailhead: From Hwy. 101, take Sir Francis Drake Blvd. 19.3 miles to the trailhead on the south side of the road. Park along the road.

Route Directions

Southern Segment: Begin on north side of Bolinas–Fairfax Rd. at junction with Ridgecrest Blvd.

3.4 Pass McCurdy Trail.

5.0 Pass Randall Trail.

9.8 Veer left on Bolinas Ridge Trail at junction with Jewell Trail. Continue on Ridge Trail for out-and back run of up to 22.2 miles, or do 11.1-mile car shuttle trip.

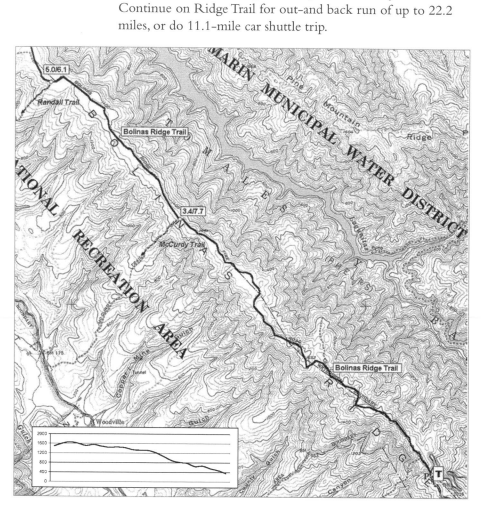

BOLINAS RIDGE, SOUTHERN SEGMENT

Northern Segment: Begin at trailhead on Sir Francis Drake Blvd.

1.0 Veer right on Bolinas Ridge Trail.

1.3 Veer right on Bolinas Ridge Trail at junction with Jewell Trail.

6.1 Pass Randall Trail.

7.7 Pass McCurdy Trail.

Continue on Ridge Trail for out-and back run of up to 22.2 miles, or do 11.1-mile car shuttle trip.

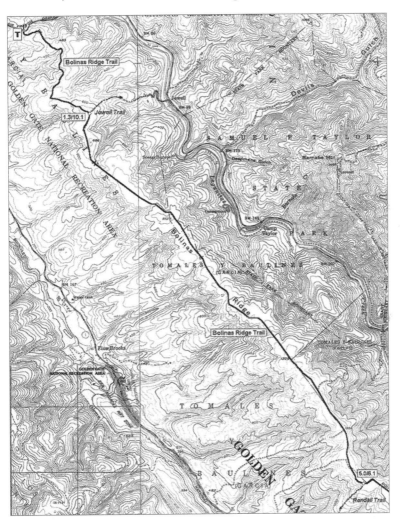

BOLINAS RIDGE, NORTHERN SEGMENT

Southern Segment: Bolinas Ridge begins at the northern reaches of Mt. Tamalpais' Tamalpa Ridge and extends northwest the length of Olema Valley and Tomales Bay. The Bolinas Ridge Trail runs from Ridgecrest Blvd. to Sir Francis Drake Blvd., near the town of Olema. A Bay Area Ridge Trail sign at the start indicates that the trail is part of the 400-mile Ridge Trail route that will eventually encircle the entire bay.

Towering coast redwoods and Douglas-fir envelop the southern end of the Bolinas Ridge Trail (the forest is so dense here that snow often remains beneath the trees for days after especially cold winter storms). Ferns and evergreen huckleberry line the wide, duff-covered trail, along with Douglas iris and milkmaids in spring.

You soon emerge in open chaparral on a hard-packed dirt and rocky surface. Manzanita, ceanothus, and scrub oak shield the coast from view. The trail rolls up and down, but mostly down, for the first 8 miles. Where redwoods yield to manzanita, views of Bolinas Lagoon and the Pacific peek through the high shrubs to the west. To the east, Pine Mountain Ridge rises above rolling hills. Turn around at McCurdy or Randall trails (at mile 3.4 or 5.0) or continue on to Sir Francis Drake Boulevard. The forest becomes less dense as you approach the northern segment of Bolinas Ridge Trail and emerge on open grasslands.

Northern Segment: The northern segment of the Bolinas Ridge Trail begins in bucolic West Marin on the pastoral ridgeline east of Olema Valley. Squeeze through the wooden cattle guard to begin the trail. On a gentle incline, the route climbs through rolling coastal rangeland, passing gullies where bay laurel and Douglas-fir trees grow in thick clumps. During the summer and fall, these vibrant evergreen trees contrast with golden grassy slopes; in spring, glossy yellow buttercups dot green pastures. Behind you, the elongated blue finger of Tomales Bay cuts between the Point Reyes Peninsula and the mainland, and the folds of volcanic Black Mountain rise in the northeast. You have views southwest of Olema Valley and densely wooded Inverness Ridge, where a thick fog bank often peeks over the top.

The trail grows wilder as it continues on a fairly level and exposed course. Fewer cows graze the hillsides (although you'll go through a number of cattle gates or stiles along this stretch of the trail) and coyote bush and blackberry line the trail's edges. Small

110 Trail Runner's Guide San Francisco Bay Area

ponds surrounded by reeds occupy low depressions, and Douglas-fir, oak, and bay laurel grow where the hills ripple together. After about 4 miles the trail climbs fairly steeply.

Beyond the junction with the Randall Trail (6.1 miles), the open pastures give way to Douglas-fir and redwood forest. See the above description of the southern segment.

Alternate Routes

From either starting point, a trip down the Jewell Trail into Samuel P. Taylor State Park is an optional route, as long as you have someone (or a car) meet you there. The Shafter Trail, although it also drops from the ridge into Samuel P. Taylor State Park, is not a good route, as there is no bridge over Lagunitas Creek and fording the creek could be hazardous.

To do an 8-mile loop into Olema Valley from Bolinas Ridge, combine the Randall and McCurdy trails with the Olema Valley Trail (part of Point Reyes National Seashore) and the Bolinas Ridge Trail. Park on Highway 1 at the Randall Trailhead, 5 miles south of Olema. The Randall Trail begins on the east side of the highway. After 1.5 miles, turn right on the Bolinas Ridge Trail and continue for 1.6 miles. Turn right again to descend the (very steep) McCurdy Trail to Highway 1. Cross the highway to pick up the Olema Valley Trail and turn left to return 2.9 miles to your car.

Trail Notes

• Fire trail
• Wide and smooth; a few muddy spots in the rainy season
• Dogs on leash
• Bikes allowed
• Horses allowed
• No toilets or water
• No fees
• Busy on weekends, especially popular with mountain bikers

See Bear Valley Loop (Run 17) or Alpine Lake Traverse (Run 11).

Nature Notes

Pastoral Olema Valley lies in the trough of the San Andreas fault, which runs the length of the valley, from Bolinas Lagoon to Tomales Bay. The movement of the fault formed both bodies of water; the mismatched hills on both sides of the valley also indicate the presence of the fault—low, rolling grasslands to the east, and a high, thickly vegetated ridge to the west.

POINT REYES NATIONAL SEASHORE

The wing-shaped Point Reyes peninsula clings to California's northern coast just north of San Francisco. In form and position, the peninsula appears unique, and it does, in fact, boast an intriguing history and an unusually diverse collection of plants and animals.

Geologic Story

Perhaps the most significant feature of the peninsula, in that it is largely responsible for its unique character, is the San Andreas fault zone—a collection of faults about a mile and a half wide that includes the major San Andreas. Bisecting Bolinas Lagoon and Tomales Bay at the southern and northern reaches of the peninsula, the San Andreas fault zone cuts through Olema Valley and separates the Pacific Plate, on which the Point Reyes peninsula lies, and the North American Plate, the mainland's plate.

The Point Reyes peninsula is a migrant to the Northern California coast—and a temporary one, at least in geologic time. Geologists believe that the peninsula formed about 80 million years ago, hundreds of miles south of where it lies today. Over the subsequent millennia, the peninsula crawled northward at an average rate of about 2 inches per year. In another few million years, Point Reyes may be in Alaska. Some of this movement is what geologists call "creep"—slow, intermittent movement that we are not aware of. However, most of the journey occurs literally in leaps and bounds, as when the peninsula moved 20 feet in the 1906 San Francisco Earthquake on the San Andreas fault.

One unusual feature of Point Reyes is the granitic rock that composes the bulk of the peninsula. This pinkish-grey rock, peppered with black grains, distinguishes the peninsula from the north Coast Range along California's mainland. From Tomales Point, at the northern tip of the peninsula, to Mt. Wittenberg, about halfway down the length of the land mass, the granitic basement rock is exposed. South of Mt. Wittenberg, marine sediments that accumulated on the peninsula during its ocean journey overlay the granite. The peninsula's topography has been shaped by repeated uplifting and submersion, as well as by weathering and erosion, as it moved up the coast.

Natural Diversity

The geologic story of Point Reyes is only one unique aspect of this vibrant peninsula. The dramatic coastal cliffs, pastoral grasslands, lush forests, and fragrant chaparral are home to a remarkable range of

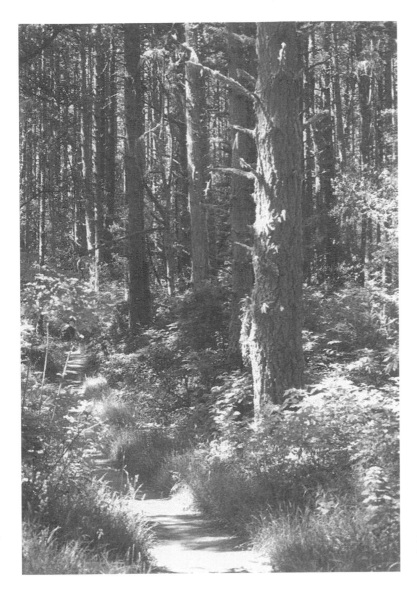

Douglas-firs along
the Old Pine Trail
(Run 17)

plants, birds, and other animals. More than 45% of the bird species found in North America visit Point Reyes at some point during the year. It is home to more than 850 flowering plant species, including more than 60 plant species not found anywhere else in Marin County.

Freshwater and saltwater marshes border northern beaches; beach grasses, lupine, and evening primrose support sandy dunes along the coast. Inland from the immediate shore, plants characterized as coastal scrub—coyote bush, sagebrush, sticky monkeyflower, and poison oak, among others—grow on the western slope of Inverness Ridge and parts of the northern peninsula. Bishop pine and Douglas-fir forests cover Inverness Ridge from Tomales Bay to Bolinas Lagoon. European annuals replace native bunchgrasses in coastal prairie and grassland; but in spring, showy native wildflowers like checkerbloom, blue-eyed grass, sun cups, buttercups, meadow foam, and ithuriel's spears cover the grassy knolls.

Windswept coastal dunes and bishop-pine-covered ridges dominate the northern reaches of the peninsula. Stark cliffs drop to smooth beaches, and wildlife populates estuaries and lagoons. Inverness Ridge, the spine of the peninsula, stands between the coast and Tomales Bay in the north and pastoral Olema Valley in the south. Mt. Wittenberg rises as the highest point on the ridge at 1407 feet and offers an overview of the peninsula. Old ranch roads and single-track trails between pastoral Olema and Bear valleys and the coast provide numerous routes over the densely forested ridge.

Climate The Bay Area's characteristic warm, dry summers and cool, rainy winters prevail on Point Reyes. The peninsula receives the most rainfall between December and March. From April through October very little precipitation falls in the form of rain. However, thick, drippy fog, heaviest in July, August, and September, moistens the lush forests along Inverness Ridge and frequently blankets the beaches and headlands in summer. Just a few miles inland, Olema Valley usually remains bathed in sunshine and warmth. Summer temperatures can differ by 20 degrees between the inland valleys, sheltered by Inverness Ridge, and the cooler coastal areas. Heavy winds, usually strongest in the spring, often beat on the peninsula, especially along the coast. Seek out Point Reyes' trails for cool relief on hot summer days, or for dazzling views on clear and crisp winter days. Bring layered clothing and be prepared for dramatic changes in temperature year round.

Trails More than 140 miles of trails traverse an extraordinary range of habitats at Point Reyes National Seashore. Most are well signed and generally easy to follow, although you should be aware that the mileage posted on trail signs is not always correct.

Official park maps divide the peninsula into two districts. In this book, the featured trails are concentrated in the South District. One North District trail in particular, not included in this book because of the long drive to reach it and its unpredictable wind and fog, is well worth visiting: the dramatic coastal bluffs of the Tomales Point Trail are showered with wildflowers in spring, and on a clear day, this 9.4-mile out-and-back route affords spectacular views of the coast, Tomales Bay, and Bodega Head.

The Point Reyes National Seashore is home to fragile and unique habitats. Take great care not to disrupt the natural environment.

What You'll Find

Rangers at the Bear Valley visitor center at park headquarters (415-464-5100) can answer questions about trails and conditions, and provide you with free maps and information sheets. The center also has an informative exhibit about Point Reyes natural history. The center's hours are Monday through Friday 9 AM to 5 PM, and Saturday and Sunday 8 AM to 5 PM.

Dogs are not allowed on trails, in campgrounds, or at most beaches in Point Reyes National Seashore. Dogs on a leash no longer than 6 feet are allowed the following beaches: Limantour (south of the parking lot), Kehoe, Palomarin, and Point Reyes North and South. Bikes are permitted on some old ranch roads. Horses are allowed on most trails in the park's South District—see individual runs for specific details.

15

PALOMARIN COAST
AND RIDGE

This diverse loop visits exposed coastal bluffs, shaded Douglas-fir forests, and peaceful ridgetop meadows, and takes in exhilarating views. These are wide, well-signed, and easily negotiable trails, although at some times of year, fallen tree branches and sticks demand that you watch your step. The open bluffs offer no protection from the elements—dress accordingly to insulate yourself from sun, wind, or fog.

Distance	11.2 miles
Time	1.5–2.75 hours
Type	loop
High Point/Low Point	1359′/189′
Difficulty	strenuous
Use	light
Maps	Point Reyes National Seashore South District trail map at visitor center
Area Management	Point Reyes National Seashore, National Park Service

Trailhead Access Hwy. 1, at 4.5 miles north of Stinson Beach and 9 miles south of Olema, turn west at the often unsigned Bolinas turnoff. Continue 1.7 miles to Mesa Rd., and turn right. Mesa Rd. ends at the Palomarin Trailhead.

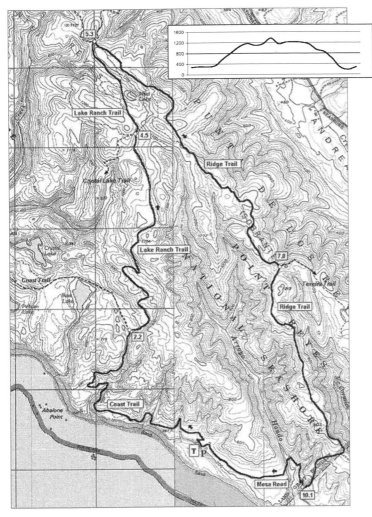

PALOMARIN COAST AND RIDGE

Begin on **Coast Trail** at the northwest end of Palomarin trailhead parking lot.

Route Directions

2.2 Turn right on **Lake Ranch Trail**.

4.5 Pass Crystal Lake Trail.

5.3 Turn right on **Ridge Trail**.

7.8 Pass Teixeira Trail.

10.1 Turn right on **Mesa Rd**.

Three trails combine to create this route: from the coast, you'll climb to the top of Inverness Ridge and then head south along the ridge to return. The loop finishes with a 1-mile stint on Mesa Road, the dirt road you drove on to reach the trailhead.

You begin on the Coast Trail just north of Palomarin Beach. The wide trail follows an open bluff coated with dense scrub. Coyote bush releases its distinct spicy fragrance, accompanied by wild cucumber and morning glory; sticky monkeyflower, Indian paintbrush, and bush lupine add bright spots of color when in bloom.

The trail sweeps up the coastline, in and out of wide gullies cut by small streams. Cow parsnip, iris, buttercups, blackberry, and ferns enliven the moist hillside ravines. You'll have excellent views of the coast on this exposed route: Bolinas Point lies behind you to the south, and to the north the coastline stretches to Abalone and Double points. Waves crash onto the narrow, pebbly beach at the foot of steep cliffs.

You soon begin a brief switchback up a dry slope and leave the coast behind. Young Douglas-firs encroach on both sides and will soon turn this open stretch into a shaded one. In spring, bright-green new growth extends from the branch tips. As you near the ridgetop, the trail narrows; high slopes shade the otherwise exposed trail, and it is strewn with small rocks.

After a short level section, you leave the Coast Trail about a half mile before Bass Lake on the clearly marked Lake Ranch Trail. Wide and grassy, the trail was once a farm road, and two distinct ruts are still visible. The vegetation is more moist and lush here than on the immediate coastal bluffs. Cow parsnip intersperses large stands of coffeeberry, leaves hang delicately from abundant hazelnut bushes, and thimbleberry, blackberry, and wild cucumber grow along the trail. Poison oak is abundant, although the trail is wide enough that you can avoid it.

Your route climbs gently to the ridge on wide switchbacks. The soft dirt trail is alternately exposed and shaded, and allows great views of the Pacific between mossy Douglas-fir branches. Fog is a frequent visitor to these coastal hillsides and keeps the forest moist. Seasonal storms bring high winds, and small branches or needles sometimes litter the trail, making footing difficult. Coffeeberry, evergreen huckleberry, elderberry, and ferns create a rich understory and a strong evergreen fragrance fills the air. Oak and fir trees encircle a serene meadow that interrupts the forest. At Mud Lake, the trail descends and wraps around the marshy pond's northwest shore, where a grassy, poppy-covered hillside meets the lake.

After turning on the Ridge Trail—at first a singletrack and then a wide trail—you head southeast along the crest of forested Inverness Ridge for about 4 miles. Sunlight spills through Douglas-fir in patches, and ferns carpet the ground. Vibrant green moss lines the soft trail, cluttered with small branches. Mud sometimes oozes across the trail, but you can avoid the worst of it.

Once you pass the Teixeira Trail, the ocean's presence becomes tangible in the subtly changing vegetation and salty breeze: poison oak reappears, milkmaids line the trail, cow parsnip and wild cucumber reclaim prominence, and sticky monkeyflower mingles with elderberry and huckleberry. The wind picks up and you pass into a different landscape: small, bushy Douglas-fir, open swards of grasses, and bright-orange springtime poppies line the trail. You begin to descend gently, and views of the coast periodically peek through trees, tall bush lupine, and coyote bush. To the east, densely forested Olema Ridge slopes toward the town of Bolinas. You can see Bolinas Lagoon and Bolinas Ridge in the distance.

As the descent steepens, you see waves crashing against the coastline. Watch out for abundant poison oak. After a brief steep downhill, from which you see Mesa Road winding toward Palomarin, you arrive at the open dirt road. Surprisingly rich vegetation lines the road—iris, ceanothus, and thimbleberry—and buckeye and bay laurel grow in the riparian ravine. As you return to the trailhead, enjoy the great coastal views beyond the dense coastal scrub on the bluffs.

Alternate Routes

For a shorter run, instead of branching off on the Lake Ranch Trail, continue on to Bass Lake on the Coast Trail. An out-and-back run to Bass Lake is 5.2 miles. Another option is to continue beyond Bass Lake to Alamere Falls at the coast (8.0 miles out-and-back).

Trail Notes

- Old ranch roads and singletrack trails
- Mostly wide, some narrow spots on Ridge Trail; debris litters Lake Ranch and Ridge trails; Lake Ranch and Ridge trails can be muddy during the rainy season, but not impassable
- No dogs
- No bikes
- Horses allowed
- Toilets at trailhead

- No water
- No fees
- The trail to Bass Lake is well traveled, especially on warm weekends, but you'll see few people on the Lake Ranch and Ridge trails

🍴 The town of Bolinas hosts two small stores with snacks to tide you over before your next meal. Try the small natural foods store behind the community center for homemade soups, delicious cookies, bins full of tasty snacks, juices, and more. Or visit the general store on the main drag.

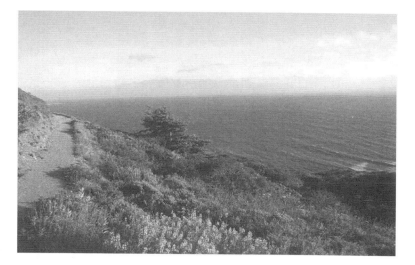

Lupine along the
Coast Trail

16

OLEMA VALLEY
TO THE COAST

Climb singletrack trails from the Five Brooks Trailhead through Douglas-fir forest to open coastal bluffs, and stretch your legs on old, smooth ranch roads on your return. The transition from forested ridge to open coast is the real highlight of this run. Views of Wildcat Lake and the eerie forest at Firtop are also captivating.

Distance	10.8 miles
Time	1.5–2.75 hours
Type	semi-loop
High Point/Low Point	1239′/258′
Difficulty	strenuous
Use	light
Maps	Point Reyes National Seashore South District trail map at visitor center
Area Management	Point Reyes National Seashore, National Park Service

From Hwy. 1, at 3.4 miles south of Olema and 5.0 miles north of the turnoff to Bolinas, turn west on a dirt road to the Five Brooks Stables and trailhead. Park in gravel lot at the end of the road. **Trailhead Access**

NOTE: The distances on official park signs on this route may not always be correct. Use the signs for directional purposes rather than distances.

Begin at Five Brooks Trailhead.

0.2 Turn right on **Stewart Trail.**

1.0 Turn right on **Greenpicker Trail.**

2.8 Turn right again to stay on signed Greenpicker Trail.

3.5 Veer right to continue on Greenpicker toward Glen Trail.

4.5 Turn left on **Glen Camp Loop Trail,** signed 0.1 MILE TO GLEN TRAIL.

4.6 Stay straight on **Glen Trail.**

4.7 Turn right on **Coast/Glen Spur South.**

5.1 Veer left on **Coast Trail.**

6.0 Turn left on **Stewart Trail.**

6.5 Pass Glen Trail.

7.0 Pass Old Out Rd. Continue on Stewart Trail to return to trailhead.

**About the
Trail**

This route combines five trails for a dramatic loop through classic Point Reyes scenery. You may encounter poison oak when the singletrack Greenpicker and Ridge trails are overgrown, but stinging nettle is more likely to be a hazard. Be prepared for heat or fog on the exposed trails near the coast.

The Five Brooks Trailhead on Highway 1 is a convenient starting point. The nearby stables may make the trailhead seem overrun by horses, but they aren't a significant presence once you are on the trails, other than for a few muddy spots worsened by their hoof prints, and some occasional piles of excrement.

The wide Stewart Trail begins along a small mill pond and soon climbs gently through a lush forest of Douglas-fir, hazelnut, bay laurel, and big-leaf maple, with ferns and poison oak as vibrant undergrowth. You leave the old ranch road for the Greenpicker Trail, a singletrack path. Although steeper than Stewart, the moderate incline on Greenpicker occasionally abates, allowing you to catch your breath. The trail is shorter and more interesting than Stewart. Dense huckleberry bushes arch over the trail, and cow parsnip, blackberry, and sword ferns crowd the edges of the path.

As you near Firtop, the trail widens and enters a tunnel of Douglas-fir. The lush understory disappears, brown trunks stretch to towering heights, and dry needles cushion the trail. Beyond Firtop

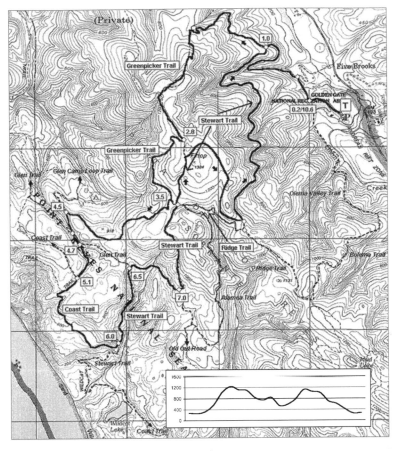

OLEMA VALLEY TO THE COAST

the vegetation returns. You descend through a quiet forest that is a vivid collage of green in spring. Subtle changes in the vegetation indicate the proximity of the coast—coyote bush becomes more frequent, often joined by wild cucumber.

After several junctions you join the Coast Trail—a narrow, exposed path that is bordered by young Douglas-fir, coyote bush, blackberry, and grasses. The blue-green ocean spreads below you, glistening in the sun or fading into fog. You will welcome the cooling coastal breeze on hot days, although it is chilling on foggy days. Smells of the ocean and fragrant coastal scrub are pungent. You will likely meet few people on this section of the trail, and may feel as though you're on the edge of the world. Wildcat Lake lies below on coastal bluffs, and to the south Double Point reaches into the Pacific at Alamere Falls (see Palomarin Loop, Run 15). You descend a wide, smooth trail bordered by lupine, coffeeberry, and morning glory.

Before you reach the coast, turn left on the Stewart Trail and head back up the ridge on the wide, smooth trail (a moderate climb of 900 feet from the coast to Firtop). Bay laurel, young Douglas-fir, coyote bush, chamise, wild cucumber, sticky monkeyflower, and cow parsnip border this exposed uphill. As you near the ridgetop, the remains of pavement reveal the trail's history as an old ranch road that was improved by the army during World War II.

To shorten your route slightly, turn right on the singletrack Ridge Trail where it meets the Stewart Trail, and detour around the southwest side of Firtop. Overgrown vegetation and mud seasonally mottle the trail, but it is a fun alternative to the wide Stewart Trail. You rejoin the Stewart Trail after only 0.5 mile. For the remainder of the run you descend gently on the shaded Stewart Trail, with views across Olema Valley to Bolinas Ridge and volcanic Black Mountain beyond.

Alternate Routes   Like other Point Reyes routes, this run presents several options, depending on the length, difficulty, and terrain you want.

For a shorter loop of 6.8 miles, climb Inverness Ridge on the Greenpicker Trail, skirt Firtop, and join the Ridge Trail at the next junction. Follow the Ridge Trail 1.2 miles to the Bolema Trail, where you turn left and begin a gradual descent 1.1 miles to the Olema Valley Trail. Another left and 1.2 miles more, and you're back at the trailhead. This route is mostly shaded and combines the singletrack Greenpicker and Ridge trails with the wider Stewart, Bolema, and Olema Valley trails, whose widths are a welcome relief from the sometimes overgrown singletracks.

If coastal views entice you to hit the beach, turn right on the Stewart Trail from the Coast Trail for a 0.7-mile detour to Wildcat Camp and Beach.

If you can arrange a car-shuttle, leave a car at the Bear Valley Trailhead, and follow the first part of the above route. When you reach the Glen Camp Loop Trail from the Greenpicker Trail, turn right and follow it to the Bear Valley Trail—total 9.4 miles. For another car-shuttle trip, follow the Coast Trail all the way to the Palomarin Trailhead (see Palomarin Run 15).

- Singletrack and fire trails
- The Greenpicker and Ridge trails are narrow in spots and over-grown with vegetation in late winter and spring; roots and debris create obstacles. Muddy during and just after the rainy season—the mud is worsened by horses
- No dogs
- Bikes on Stewart and Olema Valley trails, and the Glen Camp Loop Trail as far as Glen Camp
- Horses allowed on all trails from Five Brooks
- Toilets, water, and picnic tables at trailhead
- No fees
- The trailhead may seem crowded, but as with many trailheads, people seem to disappear once you're on the trail. The farther from the trailhead, the fewer people will you encounter, even on warm spring weekends (an ideal time of year at Point Reyes).

Bolinas or Point Reyes Station—see Palomarin (Run 15) and Bear Valley Loop (Run 17).

The San Andreas fault cuts directly through the shallow trough of Olema Valley. Movement along the fault formed the bays that lie at both ends of the valley, Tomales Bay and Bolinas Lagoon. Fault zones often create out-of-the-ordinary topography, and Olema Valley is no exception. Pine Gulch and Olema creeks demonstrate the complex drainage patterns characteristic of fault zones: the creeks run parallel to each other through the valley, separated by only about 1500 feet, but they flow in opposite directions; Pine Gulch empties into Bolinas Lagoon in the south and Olema Creek flows north to Tomales Bay. Also typical of fault zones are the small lakes or "sag ponds" that spring up along Olema Valley's floor. Olema Valley's jumbled topography, exemplified in its uplifted and folded hills and ridges, is yet another feature that reveals the existence of the San Andreas fault in the valley.

17

BEAR VALLEY LOOP

Shaded singletracks climb through a lush forest from Bear Valley to Inverness Ridge, then travel the ridgeline beneath towering Douglas-fir with views of the coastline. The wide, smooth trail through Bear Valley lets you stretch your legs as you follow the creek back to the trailhead.

Distance	6.8 miles
Time	1–1.75 hours
Type	semi-loop
High Point/Low Point	1122′/105′
Difficulty	moderate
Use	moderate
Maps	Point Reyes National Seashore South District trail map at visitor center
Area Management	Point Reyes National Seashore, National Park Service

Trailhead Access From Hwy. 1 northbound in Olema, turn left on Bear Valley Rd., 0.1 mile north of the junction with Sir Francis Drake Blvd. Continue 0.5 mile to the visitor center road; turn left and go 0.2 mile to a large paved parking area. The trailhead is at the far end of the dirt parking lot, beyond the paved lot.

From Hwy. 1 southbound, just past Point Reyes Station, turn right on Sir Francis Drake Blvd. Go 0.7 mile to Bear Valley Rd., where you turn left and continue 1.7 miles to the visitor center road. Turn right and go 0.2 mile to a large paved parking area. The trailhead is at the far end of the dirt parking lot, beyond the paved lot.

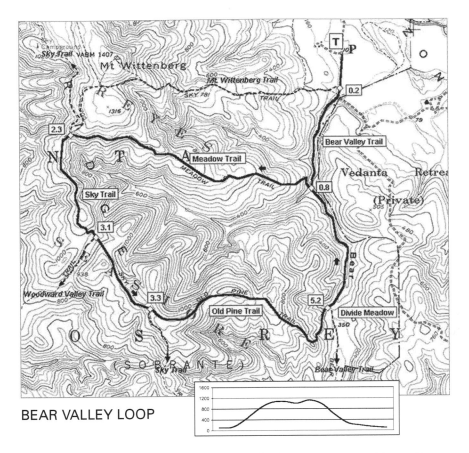

BEAR VALLEY LOOP

Begin on **Bear Valley Trail** at southern end of visitor center parking lot.

Route Directions

0.2 Pass Mt. Wittenberg Trail.

0.8 Turn right on **Meadow Trail.**

2.3 Turn left on **Sky Trail.**

3.1 Pass junction with Woodward Valley Trail.

3.3 Turn left on **Old Pine Trail.**

5.2 Turn left on **Bear Valley Trail** at Divide Meadow.

6.0 Pass Meadow Trail.

About the Trail

Many trails converge in the Bear Valley area. On this loop, you'll follow four well-signed trails, but you can customize your run by sampling a number of alternate routes.

The wide, well-graded Bear Valley Trail, shaded by alders, parallels the ravine of Bear Valley Creek. After less than a mile, you leave the level trail to ascend Inverness Ridge on the Meadow Trail, and climb steeply through a lush coastal forest. The slow pace that this grade imposes allows you to appreciate the diverse vegetation: Douglas-fir rising above tanbark oak, delicate hazelnut, and musky California bay laurel; chain fern, evergreen huckleberry, thimbleberry, and gooseberry on the forest floor. In an open meadow lined with Douglas-fir, you have views to the east (back the way you came) of Bolinas Ridge and distant Mt. Tamalpais.

You head toward the ocean on the rolling, ridgetop Sky Trail through a towering Douglas-fir forest with a rich understory of Douglas iris, western sword fern, red elderberry, and evergreen huckleberry. Light green moss drips from the fir branches. The spectacular Point Reyes coastline spreads before you, and you may be able to discern some vestiges of the 1995 Vision Fire on the coastal slopes.

On a gentle descent along the Old Pine Trail you pass another small meadow, surrounded by high trees. The towering ridgetop forest gives way to lower bushes of huckleberry and elderberry that crowd the trail. You meet the Bear Valley Trail at Divide Meadow, where the smooth path offers your legs a welcome stretch after the singletrack downhill. Follow the wide, shaded trail back to the visitor center.

Alternate Routes

The Bear Valley Trailhead offers a multitude of route combinations; most all of them are exceptional runs. In a place this spectacular, it's hard to go wrong. Experiment a little to tailor a run to your desires.

If you're looking for a shorter run, climb the Mt. Wittenberg Trail and return via the Meadow Trail. (Be forewarned that the Mt. Wittenberg Trail is the steepest route up the ridge—the Meadow and Old Pine Trails are more gradual.)

An out-and-back run to Divide Meadow on the Bear Valley Trail makes for a fairly level run (3.2 miles).

If you want to taste the salt air, follow the Bear Valley Trail all the way to Arch Rock (8.2 miles round trip). Another option to extend the featured route: continue on the Sky Trail to Baldy Trail, or even to the Coast Trail, and pick up the Bear Valley Trail to return to the trailhead (8.9 miles or 10.4 miles).

Trail Notes

- Bear Valley Trail is a wide dirt road; others are singletracks
- Some root and rock obstacles; some mud in the rainy season, especially at beginning of Meadow Trail

- No dogs
- Bicycle traffic can be heavy on weekends on Bear Valley Trail; other trails closed to bikes
- Horses allowed on all trails except on weekends and holidays
- Restroom at visitor center and in parking lot; toilet at Divide Meadow on Bear Valley Trail
- Water at visitor center
- No fees
- Helpful rangers at the visitor center can answer any questions; maps available; exhibits on the natural history of Point Reyes

The delightful town of Point Reyes Station on Highway 1 offers several spots to pick up a treat before or after a run. The Bovine Bakery whips up a delicious array of sweets, as well as breads, sandwiches, and pizzas. Sample the light buttermilk scones, sumptuous cookies, or rich peanut butter-chocolate chip brownies. The bakery is an espresso-free establishment, so warm up with regular coffee or chai tea.

For a full meal, try one of the town's many restaurants and cafes. For a picnic or snack on-the-run, you can find something to go at the good-sized Palace Market (on Highway 1, across from the bakery).

Nature Notes

If you look northwest from the Sky Trail on Inverness Ridge, you'll see a forest of burnt trees that stretches toward the coast. In 1995, 12,354 acres of land surrounding Mt. Vision were enveloped by a fire that burned 45 homes and more than 10 percent of Point Reyes National Seashore—from Limantour Beach south to Kelham Beach.

The only obvious remnants of the fire are the charred tree trunks. What isn't so obvious is that the vibrant growth that now coats the area is also a result of the fire. Fire is an essential part of the life cycles of many plants, and some literally depend on fire for survival. For instance, bishop pine and redwood seeds require intense heat from fire to burst out of their thick coats. Fire clears the forest floor of competing plants and allows the seedlings of bishop pines, redwoods, and Douglas-fir to thrive under more direct sunlight. Burned organisms release nutrients in the form of minerals, and seedlings grow vigorously in the highly fortified soil. Likewise, many annual wildflowers flourish after fire, adding vivid splashes of color to the regenerating thicket.

Fault zones often cause unusual drainage patterns, as is the case in Bear Valley. Bear Valley Creek, which borders the Bear Valley Trail from Divide Meadow to the trailhead, flows north—the opposite direction of Coast Creek, which runs west of Divide Meadow along the trail to the ocean.

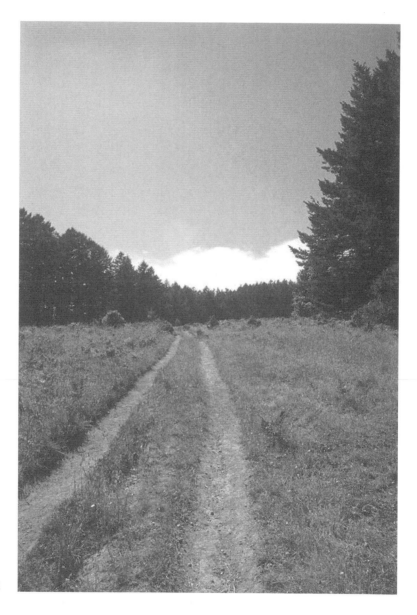

Meadow Trail

SAMUEL P. TAYLOR STATE PARK

Tucked in the rolling hills of West Marin, Samuel P. Taylor State Park extends across 2700 acres of grasslands, creekside redwoods, and mixed oak and bay laurel forests. Lagunitas Creek and several tributaries run through the park, and are important spawning streams for coho and steelhead salmon (see **Nature Notes** for Barnabe Mountain Loop, Run 18). Bolinas Ridge, east of the park, often protects these hills from coastal weather patterns, and the park is likely to be sunny when fog hangs near the coast. On hot days, the deep redwood forests offer a cool refuge.

Singletrack and fire trails traverse Samuel P. Taylor along Devils Gulch and Lagunitas creeks and up to Barnabe Mountain. You can choose from level, moderate, or steep routes.

What You'll Find

Runners, hikers, bikers, and equestrians share the trails in Samuel P. Taylor, although bikes are restricted to paved roads and fire trails. Horses are allowed on paved roads, fire roads, and some hiking trails. Dogs on leash are allowed at campsites and on roads, but not on trails. Water, restrooms, telephones, a visitor center, and picnic tables are at the state park's main entrance ($2 parking fee), 1 mile east of the Devils Gulch trailhead.

18

BARNABE MOUNTAIN

This route to 1466-foot Barnabe Mountain climbs gradually on long switchbacks through a shady forest. On clear days, your views from the peak extend north to Tomales Bay and south to Mt. Diablo and beyond. Loop back to the trailhead on a steep descent with more great views and then wind through redwoods near Lagunitas Creek. Or opt for a gentle out-and-back.

Distance	9.6 miles
Time	1.25–2.5 hours
Type	loop
High Point/Low Point	1466´/112´
Difficulty	moderate
Use	light
Maps	none at trailhead
Area Management	Samuel P. Taylor State Park

Trailhead Access From Hwy. 101 take Sir Francis Drake Blvd. for 16.2 miles to the Devils Gulch trailhead in Samuel P. Taylor State Park, 1.0 mile past the main park entrance, on the right. Park in the gravel pullout area opposite the trailhead.

Route Directions NOTE: The distances on state park signs on this route are not always in agreement with other published books and maps. Sometimes they don't agree with themselves. Use the signs for directional purposes rather than distances.

Cross highway and walk up paved Devils Gulch Rd.

0.1 Veer right at TRAIL sign.

0.3 Turn right to cross bridge. Turn left immediately after bridge, signed to **BARNABE PEAK** (**Bills Trail** on most maps).

0.8 Veer right past turnoff to Stairway Falls.

4.0 Turn left on **Barnabe Trail**.

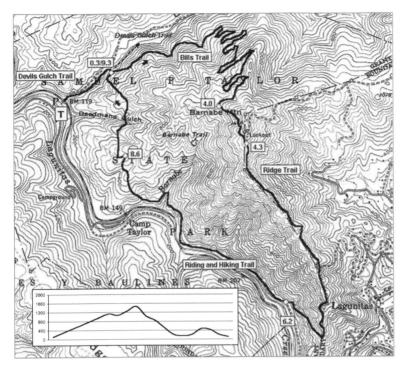

BARNABE MOUNTAIN

4.3 Turn right on **Ridge Trail.**

6.2 Turn right on **Riding and Hiking Trail**, signed to Irving Picnic Area. (From here, follow Riding and Hiking and Barnabe trails to return to Devils Gulch.)

6.9 Veer right on Riding and Hiking Trail, signed to Devils Gulch, just beyond Irving picnic area. Stay right at all junctions until Barnabe Trail.

8.6 Turn left at signed junction with **Barnabe Trail.**

9.3 Turn left to cross bridge over Devils Gulch Creek, at junction with Bills Trail; retrace steps to Sir Francis Drake Blvd.

About the Trail

Follow the paved road from Sir Francis Drake Boulevard through a forest of bay laurel, big-leaf maple, California buckeye, and alder, high above Devils Gulch Creek. After 0.1 mile, a singletrack dirt path branches right and approaches the creek; hazelnut, elderberry, and coffeeberry border the trail, and poison oak laps at your legs. You cross a wooden bridge, and on the other side begin a gradual climb out of the gulch on Bills Trail. Lush foliage thrives beneath dense tree-cover; ferns grow along the moist trail, and verdant moss cloaks bay laurel trunks. Columbine and forget-me-not are among the spring wildflowers you may see. Across Devils Gulch, open hills ripple toward the coast.

The smooth dirt trail switchbacks endlessly on a gentle grade and crosses a number of wooden bridges. As you climb higher, the trees begin to thin and grassy slopes extend into the forest cover. Bills Trail ends, and you make a final burst to the summit up the wide, steep, and exposed Barnabe Trail. Buckeye and bay laurel dot the slopes, but don't offer shade, and mugwort, cow parsnip, sticky monkeyflower, and wild cucumber line the trail.

When you reach the ridgetop, climb the last few hundred yards to the peak if you like, or pause where you are and enjoy views of Mt. Tamalpais to the southeast, Tomales Bay and the Point Reyes peninsula to the northwest, and volcanic Black Mountain almost directly north.

To loop back to the trailhead, descend on the Ridge Trail, a wide fire road. Below you, the mountain's slopes fold into forested draws, and the town of Lagunitas' residential enclaves encroach on the open rolling hills. Redwoods cover the hillside across Sir Francis Drake Boulevard, and the Kent Lake spillway sends water into Lagunitas/Papermill Creek. The Ridge Trail crosses a few stands of Douglas-fir and bay laurel, where thimbleberry and hazelnut line the trail, but this section is mostly exposed until it nears the creekbed and the Riding and Hiking Trail.

You can hear cars on Sir Francis Drake Boulevard as the trail descends steeply into the creek canyon. In spring, magnificent clarkia—red ribbons—cover a rocky hillside, accompanied by the bright blossoms of Indian paintbrush.

You join the wide, flat Riding and Hiking Trail, and after less than a mile along the creek, you reach Irving Picnic Area and veer onto a rolling singletrack beneath bay laurel and oaks. For the next mile or so, the Riding and Hiking Trail runs close to the road, although the road is mostly not visible. The trail then leaves the roadside and climbs and descends over exposed grassy hillsides and through shaded bay laurel forests to reach the Barnabe Trail. On the Barnabe Trail, you make several steep and rocky descents to return to Devils Gulch, your starting point.

To avoid the steep downhill grades on the Ridge Trail, retrace your steps from Barnabe Mountain on Bills Trail to return to the trailhead (8.6 miles out-and-back). **Alternate Routes**

The Devils Gulch Trail follows the creek on a fairly level course. Continue straight instead of turning right on the wooden bridge for an out-and-back route of about 4 miles.

Trail Notes

- Fire roads and singletrack
- Smooth dirt singletrack; steep sections on fire roads; some mud during the rainy season
- No dogs
- Bikes allowed on fire roads
- Horses allowed on fire roads and some singletrack trails
- Toilets at trailhead—continue on the paved road past the trail turnoff to two wooden toilets at the south edge of a meadow and picnic area.
- No water
- No fees at Devils Gulch

Stop in at the Lagunitas Grocery (at Sir Francis Drake Blvd. and West Cintura Avenue in Lagunitas) for a bite to eat. The deli makes milkshakes, smoothies, sandwiches, and salads. You'll also find a range of breakfast treats and espresso drinks. The grocery stocks drinks, some fruit, and other basics.

Nature Notes

The 5-mile Devils Gulch tributary of Lagunitas Creek is one of the best places in West Marin to see spawning coho (silver) salmon. After about a year in the freshwater creek of their birth, salmon migrate to the ocean to spend the next two years of their lives. Near the end of this three-year cycle, the fish return to their nascent watershed. On their way upstream, salmon focus all energy on reproduction: they no longer feed, and their bodies become tattered and scratched. Females create small depressions (redds) in the gravel on stream bottoms, where they lay their eggs; males fight each other to establish dominance and the victor fertilizes the eggs. Some salmon spawn after as few as 24 hours in freshwater, and at most, they live only 21 days after entering the stream. The dead fish contribute vital nutrients to the riparian habitat, as a source of food for animals and a nitrogen source for plants.

Coho salmon were once bountiful in West Marin creeks; historic accounts report virtual silver rivers of salmon—3,000 to 5,000 fish annually. In Devils Gulch alone, nearly 200 were counted one year. The number of salmon in the Lagunitas Creek watershed has fallen dramatically over the last 150 years. Dams, logging, road construction, fires, and gravel mining have all contributed to the destruction of salmon habitat in the watershed. Several local groups devote themselves to creek restoration, and the Marin Municipal Water District is working on a long-term restoration project to reduce sediments in the creeks and to create pools with large woody debris, in order to improve conditions for migrating salmon.

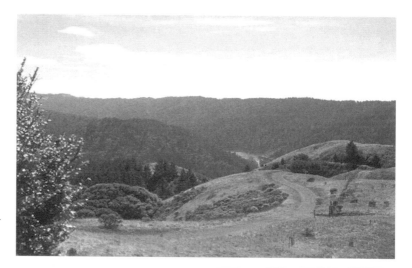

View of
Kent Lake from
the Ridge Trail

MARIN COUNTY OPEN SPACE DISTRICT

Marin County has a long tradition of environmental awareness and activism. Since the early 1900s, when development threatened land on Mt. Tamalpais, Marin residents have repeatedly banded together to preserve open space in their county. In 1972, they voted to form and fund the Marin County Open Space District (MCOSD). Since then, the district has created 32 preserves, encompassing thousands of acres. Sprinkled throughout the county, the preserves are convenient

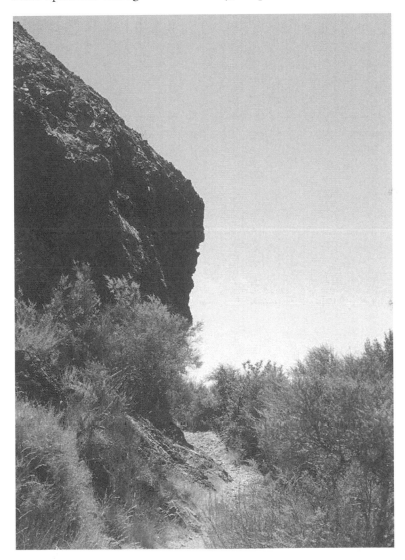

Chaparral on the Hoo-Koo-E-Koo Trail (Run 19) at Blithedale Ridge

to homes, schools, and neighborhood businesses. These open spaces protect Marin's oak-studded hills, redwood groves, wetlands, and urban wildlife from ever-encroaching sprawl, and contribute significantly to the natural spaces preserved by Marin's state and national parks and water district land.

What You'll Find

Because MCOSD policy is to minimize human impact on the preserves, you won't find water or toilets at any of the trailheads. A recognizable green sign identifies each trailhead as part of the MCOSD and lists the rules and regulations.

Dogs are allowed off leash on fire protection roads if under the direct and immediate control of a responsible person. In other areas, they must be on a 6-foot-maximum leash, and in sensitive wildlife habitats, they may be under further restrictions. Bikes are allowed on fire roads that are at least eight feet wide. They are not allowed on singletrack trails. Horses are permitted on trails and fire roads unless there are signs restricting them.

19

BLITHEDALE RIDGE

Redwood forests, fragrant chaparral, sweeping views, narrow single-tracks, expansive fire trails, steep climbs, exciting descents, fast flats—all in a 5-mile loop! This versatile low-elevation trailhead on Mt. Tamalpais' northeast side provides excellent access to the mountain's network of scenic singletracks. You can usually count on sun here when fog envelops the coast; parts of this run include exposed trails that heat up quickly.

Distance	5.4 miles
Time	0.75–1.25 hours
Type	loop
High Point/Low Point	913′/314′
Difficulty	moderate
Use	moderate
Maps	none at trailhead (see Appendix II for resources)
Area Management	Marin County Open Space District

Trailhead Access

From Hwy. 101, take Sir Francis Drake Blvd. 2.0 miles to College Ave. in Kentfield. Turn left on College Ave. and then turn right at the first stop sign onto Woodland Rd. At the next stop sign, after 0.2 mile, turn left on Evergreen Dr. Follow Evergreen for 1.0 mile to Crown Rd. and turn left. The street dead-ends after 0.2 mile. Park on the side of the road.

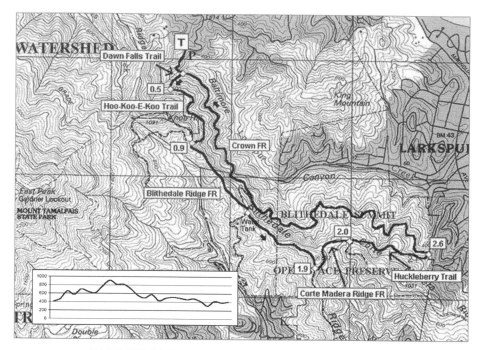

BLITHEDALE RIDGE

Route Directions

Begin on **Crown Fire Rd.** (signed as Southern Marin Line Fire Road on most maps).

0.3 Turn right on **Dawn Falls Trail.**

0.5 Turn left on **Hoo-Koo-E-Koo Trail.**

0.9 Turn left on unsigned **Blithedale Ridge Fire Rd.** Pass three unsigned side-branching trails.

1.9 Turn left on unsigned **Corte Madera Ridge Fire Rd.**

2.0 Turn left on **Huckleberry Trail.**

2.6 Turn left on **Crown Fire Rd.**

About the Trail

This featured run has some good climbs without being too taxing. While Crown Fire Road is the longest completely flat trail on Mt. Tamalpais (2.8 miles), hills aren't hard to come by in this area.

Crown Fire Road begins from a residential Kentfield neighborhood as a wide, exposed trail. Just after setting out, you pass a signpost for the Hoo-Koo-E-Koo Trail on the right. You'll meet Hoo-Koo-E-Koo again via the Dawn Falls Trail after a brief warmup on flat Crown Fire Road. Turn right on the Dawn Falls Trail, a

narrow, shaded singletrack that climbs switchbacks up a steep redwood canyon. In early spring, look for bright red and yellow mushrooms in the moist soil beneath bay laurel, ferns, evergreen
huckleberry, and tanbark oak.

Turn left on the singletrack Hoo-Koo-E-Koo Trail, a narrow trail
that angles southwest up the hillside on a gentle ascent to Blithedale
Ridge. Manzanita, madrone, bunchgrasseses, sticky monkeyflower,
and morning glory cover the dry slope, and ferns and hazelnut grow
in the shade of oak and bay laurel. In spring, look for tall purple
hound's tongues, dainty white milkmaids, the yellow stalk of star lily,
and abundant iris. Watch for rocks and roots in the trail.

On the ridgetop, exposed Blithedale Ridge Fire Road offers
wide-reaching views of Richardson Bay, Tiburon, Angel Island, and
beyond. You descend past right-branching Horseshoe Fire Road, a
connector to Old Railroad Grade and a good access trail for further
exploration of Mt. Tam. You dip into a cool and shaded redwood
canyon on Blithedale Ridge Fire Road, and pass H-Line Fire Road
on the left, a quick route back to Crown Fire Road. Stay on
Blithedale Ridge Fire Road, and shortly thereafter, pass another offshoot of H-Line Fire Road, which branches right to connect to Old
Railroad Grade.

You begin a stiff, exposed climb on Blithedale Ridge Fire Road
and are rewarded with great views when the trail tops out. Look
back the way you came to see Pine Mountain Ridge stretching to
the north. Mt. Tam dominates the foreground, a clear network of
trails traversing the slopes. You descend briefly, round a small knoll,
and turn left to descend Corte Madera Ridge Fire Road. Oak and
madrone line the exposed trail and Warner Canyon is far below on
your right.

At a multi-trail junction, you turn left on the Huckleberry Trail
and descend this singletrack to Crown Fire Road through dry chaparral and moist redwood forest. Enormous tufts of bunchgrasses send
weeping foliage down the low hillsides. Manzanita, scrub oak, toyon,
huckleberry, and madrone line rocky sections of the trail, and eroding soil makes footing difficult in places. Erosion also threatens the
soft, duff-covered dirt trail under redwoods. Choose your footing
carefully, for your own sake and for that of the delicate hillside. In
spring, pale violet iris, yellow star lily, and milkmaids line the trail,
and honeysuckle spreads its creeping foliage and pink blossoms.

Alternately level and descending, the trail is rocky and rutted in sections—watch your footing, but don't miss great views.

You leave the Huckleberry Trail and meet Crown Fire Road at its opposite end from where you began. Shadows from the high rim of the canyon cast morning and afternoon shade along the otherwise exposed trail. Big-leaf maple, bay laurel, and madrone line its edges, and in spring, the bittersweet smell of French broom pervades the air. Soon, redwoods provide more shady covering and enough moisture for lush moss to grow on hillside rocks. You pass a pump station and the H-line Fire Road intersection, and soon after that the trail begins to parallel an odd contraption—the 24-inch pipeline that transports water from the Bon Tempe treatment plant to southern Marin. Crown Fire Road becomes increasingly more exposed to the sun and heat as you near its Kentfield end and your trailhead.

Alternate Routes

So many options! This trailhead offers plenty of alternate routes for more or less distance and challenge.

The Hoo-Koo-E-Koo Trail as it continues west of Blithedale Ridge Fire Road is a short but delightful jaunt through chaparral (sweet-smelling pitcher sage and pink honeysuckle blossoms line the trail in spring). Instead of turning left on Blithedale Ridge Fire Road, cross the trail to stay on the Hoo-Koo-E-Koo Trail for 0.6 mile. A tunnel of manzanita arcs over this great singletrack. Turn right on the Corte Madera Creek Trail and climb to Hoo-Koo-E-Koo Fire Road (different from the trail). Either turn right again to follow it back to Blithedale Ridge Fire Road, or turn left and continue up the mountain to Old Railroad Grade and connecting trails.

You can also follow Blithedale Ridge Fire Road to Indian Fire Road to Eldridge Grade, which links to a network of trails on the mountain.

For a 2.7-mile loop, and to escape a major uphill section of the featured run, turn left on the H-Line Fire Road from Blithedale Ridge. Turn left again on Crown Fire Road and return to the trailhead.

Trail Notes
- Fire roads and singletrack trails
- Some narrow trails; rock and root obstacles on Hoo-Koo-E-Koo and Huckleberry trails; some eroded sections on Huckleberry
- Bikes allowed on Crown, Blithedale Ridge, and Corte Madera Ridge fire roads

- Horses allowed on Crown, Blithedale Ridge, and Corte Madera Ridge fire roads
- Dogs off-leash on Crown Fire Road (Southern Marin Line Fire Road)
- No toilets or water
- No fees
- Even on weekdays, you won't be alone on these trails; close to residential neighborhoods, they are popular with runners, hikers, and dog owners.

At the intersection of College Avenue and Woodland Road in Kentfield, the Woodlands Market offers pricey gourmet food. You'll find a deli, bakery, coffee, fresh breads, and above-average supermarket fare all for well-above-average prices.

Next to the market is Willy's Café, a popular restaurant with pleasant seating on their outdoor deck. Willy's serves breakfast—pancakes, omelettes, fresh juices, espressos—plus hearty sandwiches and other lunchtime fare.

20

MT. BURDELL

Grasslands speckled with massive oaks and decorative buckeye reach to 1558-foot Mt. Burdell. Fields of wildflowers cover the hillsides in spring, and golden grasses shimmer in summer and fall heat. This route follows some of the fire roads that crisscross the mountain's slopes—a satisfying and not-too-taxing loop that you can make more challenging by detouring to the peak. These trails are exposed and without a breeze they can be uncomfortable in hot weather.

Distance	5.2 miles
Time	0.75–1.25 hours
Type	loop
High Point/Low Point	1102′/336′
Difficulty	moderate
Use	light
Maps	none at trailhead (see Appendix II for resources)
Area Management	Marin County Open Space District

Trailhead Access From Hwy. 101 in Novato, exit at Atherton Ave./San Marin Dr. and go west on San Marin Dr. for 2.4 miles. Turn right on San Andreas Dr. Continue 0.5 mile to the MCOSD gate on the right. Park on the street.

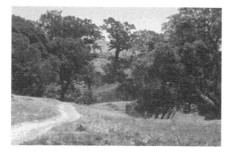

San Andreas
Fire Road

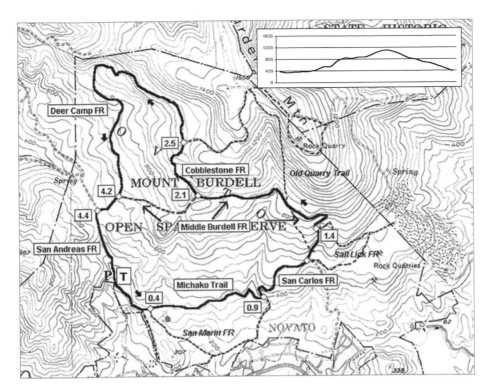

MT. BURDELL

Go through cattle guards on right of metal open-space gate. Begin on singletrack trail on right and continue right where it joins fire road. **Route Directions**

0.2 Pass San Andreas Court Fire Rd.

0.4 Go straight on **Michako Trail**. Pass wide trail that branches uphill to left.

0.9 Turn left on **San Carlos Fire Rd.**

1.2 Pass Salt Lick Fire Rd.

1.3 Pass Old Quarry Trail.

1.4 Turn left on **Middle Burdell Fire Rd.**

1.6 Pass Old Quarry Trail again.

2.1 Turn right on **Cobblestone Fire Rd.**

2.5 Turn left on **Deer Camp Fire Rd.**

4.2 Turn right on **Middle Burdell Fire Rd.**

4.4 Turn left on **San Andreas Fire Rd.**

About the Trail

To begin, take the singletrack trail on the other side of the cattle gate at the trailhead, which quickly becomes a wide fire road. The trail levels at the top of a brief climb, yielding expansive views of the town of Novato, the ridges beyond, and all the way to the tip of San Pablo Bay (where you'll often see fog creeping northward).

Continue across the open slopes to the wide, level Michako Trail. Other than two rock-strewn seasonal creekbeds, few obstacles hamper progress on the smooth trail. When you meet San Carlos Fire Road, you climb steeply into a shady oak and bay laurel forest.

You meet Middle Burdell Fire Road and turn left. A short climb brings you to a creek to the left of the trail. In spring, bright yellow monkeyflowers fill the moist area, joining year-round ferns and reeds. You enter the shade of oak and bay laurel again and continue to climb, surrounded by the strong smell of the laurel. The trail curves to the left after another cattle gate, and you now head northwest. You emerge from the trees to steep, open hills that rise to the peak, dotted with stands of oak and bay.

If you're inspired to reach Mt. Burdell's peak, take the narrow Old Quarry Trail on the right for a steep and rocky—yet beautiful—climb (see **Alternate Routes**). Otherwise, you begin a gentle descent on Middle Burdell Fire Road, watching for rocks in the trail.

Look for turkey vultures and hawks soaring overhead. You pass Hidden Lake on your left. This vernal pool is unrecognizable as a lake in summer and fall, yet it is full of water in winter and of brilliant wildflowers in spring, among them water buttercups, white forget-me-nots, and quillwort. Just past Hidden Lake you begin a steep climb on Cobblestone Fire Road. On this short hill you'll have views of open hills rolling toward Bolinas Ridge in the northwest. In spring, poppies and blue dicks cover the hills.

You leave Cobblestone Fire Road at the crest for the gentle undulations and cooling breeze on Deer Camp Fire Road. Watch for deep ruts in the trail. Large buckeyes grace these slopes, and in early spring vibrant green new growth adorns their spare branches before the long white flower spikes appear. In summer they begin to lose their leaves, and by fall, their curving branches are bare again.

Enjoy a gradual downhill all the way back to the trailhead on Middle Burdell and San Andreas fire roads.

Alternate Routes

Mt. Burdell Open Space Preserve encompasses nearly 1560 acres of open space, and the preserve's many trails and fire roads offer plenty of options to extend or shorten your run. For a 3.6-mile loop, stay on Middle Burdell Fire Road instead of taking Cobblestone Fire Road to Deer Camp Fire Road. You'll reach San Andreas Fire Road in 0.5 mile.

To climb to the peak, begin on the main route and turn right on the singletrack Old Quarry Trail from San Carlos Fire Road. The Old Quarry Trail meets the paved Ridge Fire Road after 0.7 mile. Turn right again to reach the top after 0.3 mile. Follow the rest of the featured route to return to the trailhead, or descend the single-track Mount Burdell Trail to the trailhead in Olompali State Historic Park, on the other side of the mountain (6.0 miles). You can reach the Olompali trailhead from Highway 101.

- Fire roads and singletrack
- Some rocky and rutted sections; dusty in summer, muddy in winter
- Bikes allowed on fire trails
- Horses allowed on fire trails
- No toilet or water
- No fees
- Trails are well used by hikers and equestrians.

You'll find the well-stocked Apple Market just down the road from the trailhead at San Marin Drive and San Andreas Drive.

Nature Notes

Mt. Burdell's Hidden Lake is one of the few vernal pools in Marin County. Vernal pools are small, seasonal wetlands that support a variety of unique and endangered plants and animals. In winter the pools fill with water and draw mating salamanders and toads and migrant waterfowl. The water begins to evaporate in spring and the wetlands overflow with wildflowers. Few plants have adapted to the unusual seasonal fluctuations of vernal pools; those that live in the pools are often rare species that cannot survive in other environments. In summer, vernal pools become dormant, bone-dry depressions until winter rains renew the unique cycle. Hidden Lake provides a home for 10 species of rare plants—as well as a habitat for water birds.

21

RUSH CREEK

This short route straddles two divergent habitats: the wetlands of the Petaluma River and the rolling oak woodlands of Green Ridge. This is a level course on broad fire roads and smooth singletracks. Rush Creek's proximity to Highway 101 makes it easy to get to, but the highway doesn't interfere with the peace and quiet of the natural setting.

Distance	4.2 miles
Time	0.5-1 hour
Type	semi-loop
High Point/Low Point	63´/1´
Difficulty	easy
Use	light
Maps	none at trailhead (see Appendix II for resources)
Area Management	Marin County Open Space District

Trailhead Access From Hwy. 101 in Novato, exit at Atherton Ave./San Marin Dr. and go east on Atherton Ave. for 0.1 mile. Turn left onto Binford Rd. (parallel to Hwy. 101) and go 0.1 mile to MCOSD gate and roadside parking.

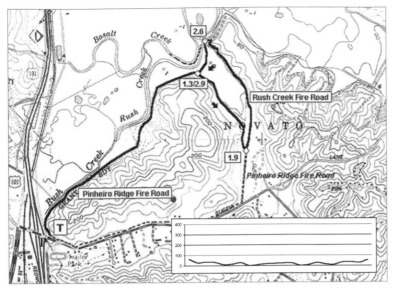

RUSH CREEK

Route Directions

Begin on **Pinheiro Ridge Fire Rd.**

1.3 Bypass singletrack coming from north; Pinheiro Ridge Fire Rd. curves right (south) to begin counterclockwise semiloop.

1.9 Cross wooden bridge and turn left (north) on **Rush Creek Fire Rd.**

2.5 Stay left where trail forks.

2.6 Turn left at junction and left again immediately at MCOSD sign.

2.7 Stay left where wider trail heads right through marsh.

2.9 Turn right on **Pinheiro Ridge Fire Rd.** and retrace route to trailhead.

About the Trail

Rush Creek's contrasting landscapes are apparent from the start of this route. Pickleweed and cattails line the wetland salt marsh on one side of the trail, and open oak-studded hills slope to meet the other side. Bay laurel, buckeye, and madrone mingle with the oaks, their branches thick with moss in winter and spring. Bunchgrasses coat the ground, interspersed with milkmaids, buttercups, and shooting stars in spring.

When the marsh is low during summer, white salt gathers along the water's edge and a brackish smell occasionally drifts over the trail. Vibrant green moss contrasts with brown grass and grey-blue water.

In fall and winter, the pickleweed turns a deep magenta. You have views of Mt. Burdell beyond the marsh.

Traffic noise dissipates as you leave Highway 101 behind, and Rush Creek seems far from the commuting cars. In a shaded segment after a slight rise, you pass a small path coming across the marsh from the north that joins your trail (you'll return on this singletrack). For now, you head southeast along the marsh, still on the Pinheiro Ridge Fire Road. This is the beginning of a counterclockwise loop around the marsh.

You cross a wooden bridge at the southernmost point of the loop and abruptly join the Rush Creek Fire Road, a wide, gravelly trail that heads north and eventually wraps around the east side of the marsh. Oak and buckeye densely coat the rolling hills to your right and California sagebrush lines the trail. Frogs chatter in the marsh, and birds, including snowy egrets, dwell near the water.

A series of left turns lead you onto the singletrack trail that crosses the marsh. Follow it to return to the Pinheiro Ridge Fire Road and retrace your steps to the trailhead.

Trail Notes • Fire trails, singletrack
- Smooth dirt; muddy patches during rainy season
- Bikes allowed
- Dogs on leash
- Horses allowed
- No toilets or water
- No fees

Cross Highway 101 to find Apple Market grocery store on the corner of San Marin and San Andreas drives, the closest food source around.

Nature Notes

Wetland and oak woodlands coexist in the 36-acre Rush Creek Open Space Preserve in the Petaluma River floodplain. You'll notice a combination of freshwater and saltwater plants growing in the marsh: those that are more salt-tolerant, such as cord grass and pickleweed, grow closest to the saltwater. Plants usually found in freshwater, such as cattails, grow in areas where the marsh is protected from the tidal flow of saltwater.

In fall, winter, and spring, Rush Creek is an ideal spot to watch shorebirds. Some of the easiest to pick out as you run by are the great egret and the snowy egret, and the white pelican.

EAST BAY TRAIL RUNS

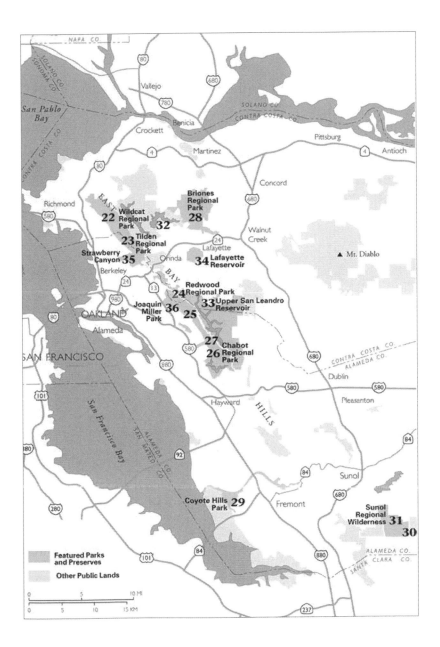

NAPA CO.

SOLANO CO.
SONOMA CO.

Vallejo

San Pablo
Bay

SOLANO CO.
CONTRA COSTA CO.

Benicia

Crockett

Pittsburg

Antioch

Martinez

Concord

Richmond

Briones
Regional
Park 28

Wildcat
22 Regional 32
Park

Walnut
Creek

Tilden
23 Regional
Park

Lafayette

Strawberry
Canyon 35

Orinda

34 Lafayette
Reservoir

▲ Mt. Diablo

Berkeley

Redwood
24 Regional Park

Joaquin
Miller 36
Park 25

33 Upper San Leandro
Reservoir

OAKLAND

Alameda

27 Chabot
26 Regional
Park

CONTRA COSTA CO.
ALAMEDA CO.

SAN FRANCISCO

Dublin

San Francisco Bay

Hayward

HILLS

Pleasanton

San Mateo Co.

Alameda Co.

Sunol

Coyote Hills
Park 29

Fremont

Sunol
Regional
Wilderness 31
30

ALAMEDA CO.
SANTA CLARA CO.

Featured Parks
and Preserves

Other Public Lands

0   5   10 MI
0   5   10   15 KM

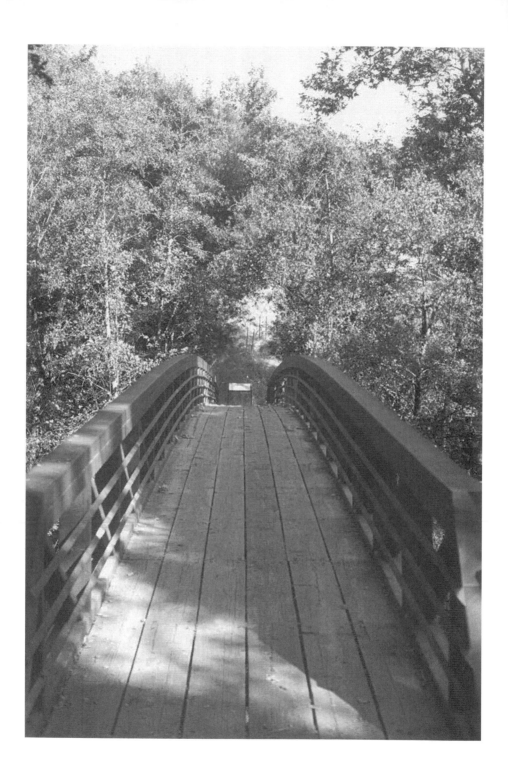

EAST BAY

LAY OF THE LAND

Directly east of the Golden Gate, across the San Francisco Bay, a broad plain spreads inland from the bay shore. The Berkeley Hills rise beyond, introducing a series of ridges and valleys that ripple eastward toward 3849-foot Mt. Diablo. The Diablo Range, crowned by Mt. Hamilton (4213 feet)—the highest peak in the Bay Area—stretches south to Pacheco Pass in Santa Clara County.

The East Bay hills form a natural barrier between the coast and the Bay Area's interior valleys. As such, they help determine the climate and habitat of the East Bay's diverse plant and animal communities. Directly across from the Golden Gate, the bay side of the Berkeley Hills receives the influence of the open ocean, and shares a marine climate with coastal areas of Marin, the peninsula, and San Francisco; the area receives the brunt of coastal fogs and breezes, as well as the benefit of moderate summer and winter temperatures.

East of the ridgeline, Contra Costa County experiences an almost entirely different climate—hotter in summer, colder in winter, and often fog-free. The South Bay, shielded from the coast by the high Santa Cruz Mountains, also experiences hotter summers, colder winters, and less fog.

The East Bay's landscape reflects its diverse climatic zones, and you'll find surprising variety within a relatively small geographic area. Redwood forests grow where fog gathers, oak trees stud open slopes, marshes and tidal zones border the bay, and grasslands cover large expanses of rolling hills.

A string of parks cap the ridgeline and dot the rolling Contra Costa County hills beyond, and a few parks rim the bay shore. Some are close to residential neighborhoods, others lie in more remote corners of the region. Most open space in the East Bay is under management of EBRPD and EBMUD, although city parks and the University of California are responsible for some smaller holdings.

Opposite page:
Bridge at
trailhead,
Sunol Regional
Wilderness
(Runs 30 & 31)

153

EAST BAY REGIONAL PARK DISTRICT

East Bay Regional Park District lands play an important role in the character of the East Bay landscape. The district's 59 parks, preserves, shorelines, and recreation and wilderness areas (92,000 acres) create an impressive collage of open space and provide valuable recreational opportunities for Bay Area residents. Most residents of Alameda and Contra Costa counties live within 15 to 30 minutes by car or bike to an East Bay Regional Park. Your next run is closer than you thought!

As East Bay cities began to expand in the early 1900s, citizens realized that the surrounding open space must be preserved. Although the East Bay Municipal Utility District owned (and thereby protected) thousands of acres of land, a 1928 decision by EBMUD to sell off surplus watershed land put the land at risk of private development. Community members mobilized to encourage the formation of a park district that would buy the surplus acres. In 1934, voters approved the creation of the East Bay Regional Park District and the surplus watershed land became its first holding, now Tilden Regional Park.

Some EBRPD parks feature short nature walks as their main attraction, like Huckleberry Botanic Regional Preserve and Sibley Volcanic Regional Preserve. Many parks, like Redwood, Chabot, Tilden, and Briones, have extensive trail networks. Altogether, in-park trails total more than 1,000 miles. In addition, a network of 29 inter-park trails link the regional parks, including the East Bay Skyline National Recreation and Bay Area Ridge trails (see Redwood and Anthony Chabot regional park runs).

What You'll Find   Check individual parks and routes for dog, bike, and horse regulations. In general, dogs are allowed off-leash on trails if under voice control. They must be on-leash in parking areas, picnic sites, and developed areas. Dogs are not allowed in creeks, wetlands, and marshes. Bikes are allowed on fire roads. Horses are allowed on most trails, although seasonal closures often make singletracks off limits for equestrians in the rainy season. Toilets and water are available in certain locations—check individual runs for specifics.

Most major EBRPD trailheads have toilets, water, and maps. The EBRPD produces brochures that include maps with detailed trail distances, information on the park's natural and human history, and contact numbers. You can usually pick up a brochure at major trailheads.

TILDEN AND WILDCAT CANYON REGIONAL PARKS

Tilden and Wildcat Canyon regional parks abut one another in the East Bay hills behind Berkeley, Albany, and El Cerrito; together they cover about 4,500 acres. Both extend from the broad valley of Wildcat Creek, Tilden to the south and Wildcat Canyon to the north. From the valley floor, the Berkeley Hills rise to the west and San Pablo Ridge to the east.

A network of trails runs through Wildcat Canyon and up and down San Pablo Ridge and the Berkeley Hills; trailheads scattered throughout the parks provide numerous start- and end-points. The parks are close to residential neighborhoods and easily accessible from East Bay communities both east and west of the Berkeley Hills. After you familiarize yourself with the featured runs, explore other routes on the trails that crisscross these parks.

What You'll Find

Tilden and Wildcat regional parks are open to dogs, bikes, horses, hikers, and runners, with certain restrictions. Check individual trails for specifics. In general, dogs are allowed off-leash if under voice control; dogs are not allowed at all in Tilden Nature Area, where the featured Wildcat Canyon run begins. Bikes are allowed on fire trails. Horses are allowed on most trails except for a cluster of hikers-only trails near Tilden Nature Area. Toilets and water are available in many locations—check individual runs for specifics.

The East Bay's clay soil turns muddy during the rainy season and can make many Tilden and Wildcat Canyon trails unpleasant. You'll encounter muddy patches on the Wildcat Canyon and Meadows Canyon trails in particular. Trails in Tilden's southern area are generally less muddy.

The Wildcat Regional Park entrance is in Richmond, but the trails are also accessible through Tilden. Tilden has several entrances and numerous trailheads. The two featured runs begin in at two different trailheads in the northern section of Tilden Park.

22

WILDCAT CANYON

Climb Wildcat Canyon's windy ridges to enjoy great views, cross exposed grassy hills, and follow a creekside trail in the unexpected riparian enclave of Havey Canyon. Mostly on wide fire trails, this run includes a 1.3-mile paved section along Nimitz Way, although you can follow a narrow dirt track next to the pavement for most of the way. Die-hard dirties will find completely pavement-free runs in the alternate routes section.

Distance	9.3 miles
Time	1.25–2.25 hours
Type	semi-loop
High Point/Low Point	1138′/382′
Difficulty	moderate
Use	light
Maps	EBRPD map at Environmental Education Center
Area Management	East Bay Regional Park District

Trailhead Access From Interstate 80 in Berkeley, take the University Ave. exit and go east. After 2.1 miles, turn left on Oxford St. Continue 0.7 mile and turn right on Rose St. Go one block to Spruce St. and turn left. Follow Spruce 1.8 miles to the three-way intersection with Grizzly Peak Blvd. and Wildcat Canyon Rd. Cross Grizzly Peak and make an immediate left on Cañon Dr. After 0.3 mile, turn left on Central Park Dr. Park in the lot, 0.1 mile beyond.

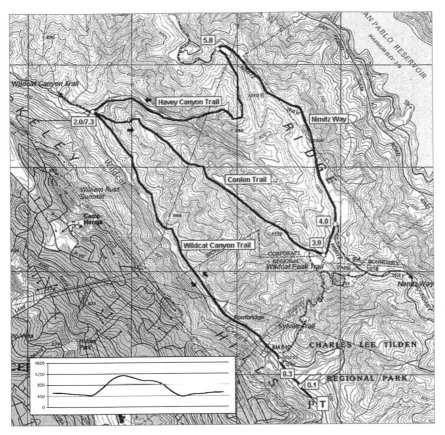

WILDCAT CANYON

Route Directions

Begin on paved road at north end of parking lot.

0.1 Pass visitor center.

0.3 Pass Jewel Lake.

2.0 Turn right at signed junction with the Conlon and Havey Canyon trails. Go through metal cattle gate. Immediately turn right again on **Conlon Trail.**

3.9 Go through cattle gate and follow trail as it curves left.

4.0 Turn left on **Nimitz Way.**

5.8 Turn left on **Havey Canyon Trail.**

7.3 Go through metal cattle gate at junction of Wildcat Canyon and Conlon trails. Turn left on **Wildcat Canyon Trail** and return to trailhead.

About the Trail This run begins at the Tilden Regional Park Environmental Education Center (EEC) and Little Farm, a popular spot for families with children. Start this route in a stand of redwoods at the far north end of the parking lot. The paved road soon turns to the wide gravel Wildcat Canyon Trail and the redwoods give way to oaks, joined by blackberry, hazelnut, currant, and red-twigged dogwood. A grove of eucalyptus extends up the hillside across the trail from Jewel Lake, where turtles sun themselves on low rocks.

The trail heads into Wildcat Canyon; to your left, Wildcat Creek flows through a riparian forest of willow, alder, creek dogwood, and bay laurel. Above the creek, the east-facing hillside is densely cloaked in coast live oak, bay laurel, big-leaf maple, and madrone. Years of grazing have converted the opposite hillside into an open slope covered with introduced annual grasses, but coyote bush is slowly gaining prominence. Introduced species such as French broom, poison hemlock, mustard, and thistle line the trail and birds flit among the grasses.

After 2 miles on the Wildcat Canyon Trail, you turn right on the Conlon Trail and begin to climb steeply. Cows graze the hillsides and raptors soar above the windy ridgetop. Your views encompass the Golden Gate, San Pablo Bay, the rolling hills of Contra Costa County, and San Pablo and Briones reservoirs. You descend briefly to the east and then head north along the open ridge on the mostly level, paved Nimitz Way.

You turn left on the Havey Canyon Trail after just under 2 miles on pavement and soon leave the expansive grasslands behind. On a gentle descent, you head into a riparian canyon, an improbable gem of lush vegetation in these exposed hills. Sweet smells of moist earth

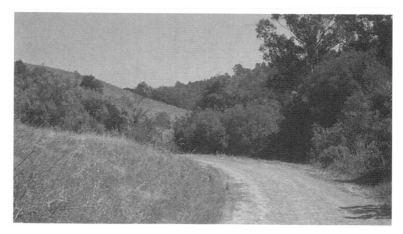

Wildcat Canyon Trail

and bay laurel mingle as you navigate the narrow trail; bunchgrasses spread under oaks on the hillside and willow and bay laurel line the creek. The bright openness of Wildcat Canyon greets you as you emerge from the riparian cover. Return to the trailhead on the Wildcat Canyon Trail.

For a shorter run, or to avoid the pavement on Nimitz Way, descend the Wildcat Peak and Sylvan trails back to the trailhead. From the Conlon Trail, instead of veering left to Nimitz Way, turn right on a wide grassy trail that leads to a bench. At the bench, go left on a singletrack to a metal gate. Pick up the singletrack Wildcat Peak Trail on the other side. Just below the peak, turn right and descend steeply at times, through a eucalyptus grove. You join the Wildcat Canyon Trail at Jewel Lake and return to the trailhead (about 5.5 miles total).

Alternate Routes

- Fire trails

Trail Notes

- Havey Canyon Trail narrow in parts; trails are rutted from cows and winter mud; extremely muddy in the rainy season
- No dogs in Tilden Nature Area; on leash on Nimitz Way; off leash in Wildcat Canyon Regional Park
- Bikes allowed on all trails except Wildcat Peak, Sylvan, and Laurel Canyon trails.
- Horses allowed on all trails except Wildcat Peak and Sylvan trails
- Restrooms in parking lot, at EEC, and at Jewel Lake
- Water near bathrooms in parking lot and at EEC
- EEC is open from 10 AM to 5 PM, Tuesday through Sunday. Maps are available out front when the center is closed.
- No fees

Berkeley's "Gourmet Ghetto" is just down the hill from Tilden Park (in the vicinity of Shattuck Avenue and Vine Street). Have a coffee at the original Peet's Coffee. Just down the street you can indulge in The Cheeseboard's delicious breads or try their mouth-watering pizza; or sit down for a hearty meal or light snack at Saul's Delicatessen. After a bite to eat, you can feed your mind at Black Oak Books next to Saul's. To get here from the trailhead, go south on Central Park Drive and then make a right on Cañon Drive. At the top of the hill, turn right onto Spruce Street. Follow Spruce to Vine Street; turn right to find Peet's; continue one more block and turn left on Shattuck Avenue for the Cheeseboard; turn right on Shattuck for Saul's.

23

MEADOWS CANYON AND
BIG SPRINGS LOOPS

This route gives you the option of an easy 3-mile loop or a longer and hillier 7-mile one. On the shorter run, you'll climb through open grasslands and return along a shaded creekbed; the longer one adds challenging climbs and panoramic views of the Bay Area.

Distance	3.1 or 7.2 miles
Time	0.5–1.75 hours
Type	loop
High Point/Low Point	1629´/538´ double loop
	969´/538´ single loop
Difficulty	easy to moderate
Use	moderate
Maps	EBRPD map at Lone Oaks trailhead
Area Management	East Bay Regional Park District

Trailhead Access From Interstate 80 in Berkeley, take the University Ave. exit and go east. After 2.1 miles, turn left on Oxford St. Continue 0.7 mile and turn right on Rose St. Go one block to Spruce St. and turn left. Follow Spruce 1.8 miles to the three-way intersection with Grizzly Peak Blvd. and Wildcat Canyon Rd. Cross Grizzly Peak and make an immediate left on Cañon Dr. After 0.3 mile, turn right on Central Park Dr. After 0.1 mile, turn left on Lone Oak Rd. and park in the lot. Walk up the paved road to the Lone Oak picnic area and trailhead.

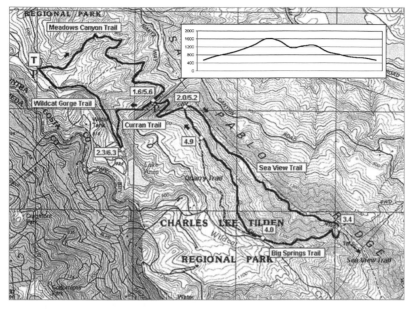

MEADOWS CANYON AND BIG SPRINGS LOOPS

Begin at metal fire trail gate just below Lone Oak Picnic Area. Veer left on **Meadows Canyon Trail** (Wildcat Gorge Trail branches right).

Route Directions

1.6 Turn right on **Curran Trail**.

Single loop: Continue straight on the **Curran Trail**.

2.3 Turn right on **Wildcat Gorge Trail**.

Double loop: From Curran Trail, veer left on spur to **Wildcat Canyon Rd**.

1.7 Pick up **Sea View Trail** across Wildcat Canyon Rd.

1.9 Pass right-branching trail to Quarry Picnic Area.

2.0 Pass right-branching Big Springs Trail.

3.4 Turn right on **Big Springs Trail**.

4.0 Cross parking lot on South Park Dr. and rejoin trail beyond metal fire trail gate.

4.1 Veer right to stay on Big Springs past Quarry Trail.

4.9 Pass Quarry Trail again.

5.2 Turn left on **Sea View Trail**.

5.6 Cross Wildcat Canyon Rd.

5.7 Turn left on **Curran Trail**.

6.4 Turn right on **Wildcat Gorge Trail**.

About the Trail   Begin this route on the Meadows Canyon Trail as it climbs gently through a wide canyon toward the rounded hills above Nimitz Way. On hot days, the sun beats down on the exposed trail, and in summer it becomes a jigsaw puzzle of rutted dirt. Coyote bush, elderberry, poison hemlock, and mustard line the trail, and on a sharp curve to the right, a small willow-lined creekbed crosses beneath.

After a short ascent through a eucalyptus grove, you reach the Curran Trail, which you can follow back to the trailhead for the 3-mile loop.

Single Loop: Look north for views of the Meadows Canyon Trail as you descend on the Curran Trail beneath tall eucalyptus. Across a deep ravine, small caves pocket a rock wall; a fence at the top is intended to detour visitors.

At Wildcat Creek, you meet the Wildcat Gorge Trail and follow it along the cool creek. On a gentle descent or level grade, the trail passes under bay, oak, and buckeye. It reaches the trailhead just after crossing a broad meadow.

Double Loop: From the Curran Trail you follow a spur trail to Wildcat Canyon Road. Across the road you join the Sea View Trail and climb steadily, at first under the cover of eucalyptus, and soon emerge on an open grassy slope. The incline abates briefly when you reach San Pablo Ridge, but you then continue up several rocky rises on the wide ridgetop trail. Along short shaded sections the trail is moist from fog drip but is otherwise mostly exposed. The Sea View Trail straddles two climates: the warm summer and cold winter temperatures of the interior valleys and the fog and cool breezes of the coast.

Along the ridgetop you have impressive views in all directions. San Pablo and Briones reservoirs nestle between bare hills, and Mt. Diablo looms above the broad valley of Contra Costa County. To the west, beyond the Berkeley Hills, the Golden Gate marks the entrance to the bay, with San Francisco and Marin on either side. Mt. Tamalpais rises like a beacon, the highest point around the bay.

A well-earned descent after the ridge's highest point leads to the Big Springs Trail, where you turn right and continue to descend on a wide rocky trail—choose your footing carefully. The trail winds through a ravine lined with grassy hills on one side and planted Monterey pines on the other. Cross the gravel parking area along

South Park Road and continue on the Big Springs Trail as it rolls up and down along the hillside below San Pablo Ridge.

You rejoin the Sea View Trail and retrace your steps down to Wildcat Canyon Road. Across the road, you begin the last leg of the loop on the Curran Trail, following the directions for the 3-mile loop.

Both of these loops stand alone as good runs, and combined they make a great hill workout with outstanding views of the Bay Area. Caveat: don't attempt the Meadows Canyon Trail in rainy seasons, unless you enjoy lugging a pound of sticky mud on the bottom of your shoes; run up and back on the Wildcat Gorge and Curran trails or skip the bottom loop altogether. You can start the upper loop from Wildcat Canyon Road, just west of Inspiration Point, where the Sea View Trail begins. **Alternate Routes**

- Wide singletrack and fire trails **Trail Notes**
- Meadows Canyon Trail often rutted from dried mud; some rocky sections on Sea View and Big Springs trails; roots along Wildcat Gorge Trail; Meadows Canyon Trail muddy during rainy season.
- Dogs off leash, under voice control
- Bikes allowed (except on Wildcat Gorge Trail during wet weather); watch for bikes on the Meadows Canyon Trail
- Horses allowed (except on Wildcat Gorge Trail during wet weather)
- Toilets and water at trailhead
- No fees

See Wildcat Canyon (Run 22).

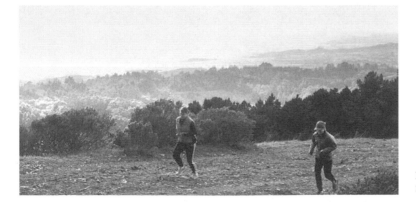

Runners on
Sea View Trail

REDWOOD REGIONAL PARK

Redwood Regional Park crowns the hills above Oakland with 1,800 acres of towering redwoods, open ridgetops, and oak and madrone forests. The park borders residential neighborhoods and is well used by runners, hikers, and mountain bikers. Runners and walkers hit the trails at first light and others come and go through the day until dark.

Redwood Canyon and its east and west ridges define the topography of Redwood Park. Redwood Creek flows through the deep canyon, bound by steep walls that rise to 1500 feet at some points. The trails in Redwood Park offer many choices for runs of varying length and difficulty along relatively flat ridgetops or into the canyon. Wide fire roads run the length of the ridges and join numerous singletrack trails that traverse the slopes below and beyond the ridges.

Redwood's trails also connect to trails in Joaquin Miller Park (see Joaquin Miller Loop, Run 36). The East Bay Skyline National Recreation and Bay Area Ridge trails run through Redwood and link the park to Anthony Chabot Regional Park (see Runs 26-27) to the south and Sibley Volcanic Preserve to the north.

What You'll Find Trails in Redwood Park are open to dogs, bikes, horses, hikers, and runners, with certain restrictions. Dogs must be leashed on the Stream Trail, where creek restoration is in progress. Bikes are allowed only on fire roads. Horses are allowed on most trails, although most singletracks are off-limits for equestrians in the rainy season. Toilets and water are available in certain locations—check individual runs for specifics.

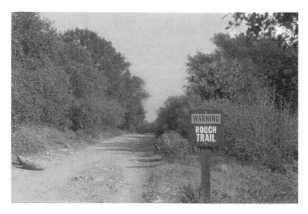

West Ridge Trail

24

WEST RIDGE LOOP

Run through cool redwood forests and cross chaparral hillsides on exposed sandstone trails. This route has great views and a good combination of climbs and descents on the park's wide fire roads.

Distance	7.8 miles
Time	1-2 hours
Type	semi-loop
High Point/Low Point	1544´/1080´
Difficulty	moderate
Use	heavy
Maps	EBRPD map at trailhead
Area Management	East Bay Regional Park District

Trailhead Access

From Hwy. 13 northbound in Oakland, take the Joaquin Miller Rd./Lincoln Ave. exit. Turn right onto Joaquin Miller Rd. Pass Joaquin Miller Park entrance. Turn left on Skyline Blvd. Pass Redwood Bowl and Moon Gate Staging Area and continue to the large parking lot at the Skyline Gate Staging Area.

From Hwy. 13 southbound, take the Joaquin Miller Rd./Lincoln Ave. exit, stay left and at a stop sign turn left onto Monterey Blvd. Immediately afterward, at the stoplight, turn left again onto Joaquin Miller Rd. Follow the directions above.

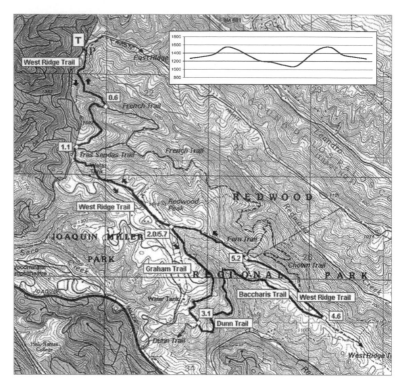

WEST RIDGE LOOP

Route Directions

Begin on **West Ridge Trail**, at far right of Skyline Gate Staging Area parking lot.

0.6 Pass French Trail.

1.1 Pass Tres Sendas Trail.

1.6 Cross paved road (to the Chabot Space and Science Center). Pass just below the center.

1.7 Cross another road to continue on West Ridge Trail.

2.0 Redwood Bowl Picnic Area. Veer right on **Graham Trail** (beginning of loop).

3.1 Turn left on **Dunn Trail.**

3.9 Pass unsigned Monteiro Trail.

4.1 Continue straight on **Baccharis Trail.**

4.6 Turn left on **West Ridge Trail.**

4.8 Pass Chown Trail.

5.2 Pass Fern Trail.

5.7 Retrace route from Redwood Bowl to trailhead.

You begin on the West Ridge Trail, a smooth, wide fire road that runs through oak, bay laurel, and an occasional stand of redwoods. Large madrones curve over the trail, and huckleberry adds its graceful foliage. The spicy scent of currants fills the air in winter. Views across the canyon of the East Bay hills and beyond to Mt. Diablo provide immediate reward. An occasional short, steep uphill interrupts gentle ups and downs as the trail hugs the ridge. You cross beneath the large glass windows and aluminum siding of the impressive Chabot Space and Science Center, where you have westward views across the bay to the San Francisco Peninsula.

About the Trail

The trail enters a redwood forest and soon passes an open glen with picnic tables. Here you join the Graham Trail, thick with duff, and begin to descend moderately through shady redwoods. The trail eventually levels and opens to terrific views of gently undulating ridges in Contra Costa County. Oaks replace redwoods in this sunny and dry section, and French broom clutters the trail—sweet-smelling and with lively yellow blossoms in spring. A deep oak-forested canyon drops to your left and you see your trail climbing on the other side. Hot and dusty in summer, this stretch is nevertheless great fun—smooth and fast.

You join the Dunn Trail and drop into the canyon you saw from above; the trail winds in and out of shady redwoods and sparse oak and madrone forest. Forget-me-nots and milkmaids bloom beneath the redwoods in spring. You traverse several gullies and then begin to climb the canyon's other side, where coyote bush, French broom, and poison oak cover the dry, exposed hillside. After a moderate climb the trail levels, passing eucalyptus groves and open swards, and crosses several potentially muddy spots in the rainy season. Enjoy this flat stretch, because shortly you turn onto the West Ridge Trail, where you climb substantially. This section of the West Ridge Trail crosses solid, embedded sandstone. Climb through eucalyptus trees to reach Redwood Bowl, where you complete the loop, and then retrace your steps along the West Ridge Trail to the trailhead.

The Redwood Bowl Picnic Area (where the West Ridge Trail meets the Graham Trail) is a good turnaround point for about a 4-mile, out-and-back run along the west ridge from Skyline Gate. This section has only a few ups and downs and avoids the long hills on the loop route.

Alternate Routes

If you want a longer route than the featured one, explore the trails that extend southeast from the Dunn Trail (Monteiro, Tate, Toyon, and Golden Spike trails) and loop back to the West Ridge Trail farther east on its ridgetop course.

Trail Notes
- Fire trails
- Wide, smooth trails; a few passable muddy spots in the rainy season
- Bikes allowed
- Horses allowed
- Dogs off leash, under voice control on this route; must be leashed on Stream and Bridle trails
- Toilet at trailhead
- Water at trailhead and at Redwood Bowl Picnic Area (2.0 and 5.8 miles)
- Heavily used park, but you can find solitude on the trails
- The smooth, wide, and relatively level West Ridge Trail is good for jogging strollers.

 Head down the hill to Montclair Village to find coffee, bagels, smoothies, delicatessens, and more. Moraga Avenue, Mountain Boulevard, and LaSalle Avenue are all good bets.

Nature Notes The land that is now Redwood Park was once a magnificent forest of *Sequoia sempervirens*. Towering in height and enormous in girth, the original coast redwoods on these hills were useful navigational landmarks for ships sailing into San Francisco Bay. In the mid-1800s, logging decimated the East Bay redwoods, and cleared Redwood Canyon of its namesake trees. Today, Redwood Park is again graced by the majestic trees; although some have reached heights of 100 feet or more, these trees are all second and third growth.

25

FRENCH TRAIL LOOP

Follow a wide, exposed trail along Redwood's west ridge and then drop into the forested canyon of Redwood Creek, a cool refuge on hot days. This route earns its difficult rating with rigorous ups and downs on the singletrack French Trail and a brisk climb back up the ridge.

Distance	6.2 miles
Time	0.75–1.5 hours
Type	semi-loop
High Point/Low Point	1542′/863′
Difficulty	strenuous
Use	moderate
Maps	EBRPD map at trailhead
Area Management	East Bay Regional Park District

Trailhead Access

From Hwy. 13 northbound in Oakland, take the Joaquin Miller Rd./Lincoln Ave. exit. Turn right onto Joaquin Miller Rd. Pass Joaquin Miller Park entrance. Turn left on Skyline Blvd. Pass Redwood Bowl and Moon Gate Staging Area and continue to the large parking lot at the Skyline Gate Staging Area.

From Hwy. 13 southbound, take the Joaquin Miller Rd./Lincoln Ave. exit, stay left and at a stop sign turn left onto Monterey Blvd. Immediately afterward, at the stoplight, turn left again onto Joaquin Miller Rd. Follow the directions above.

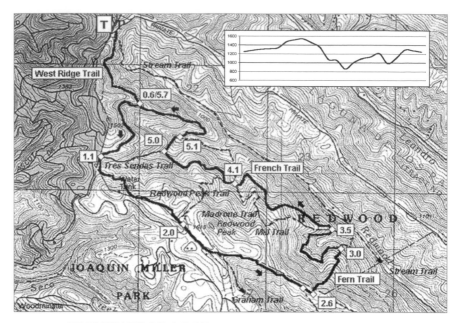

FRENCH TRAIL LOOP

Route Directions

Begin on **West Ridge Trail**, at far right of Skyline Gate Staging Area parking lot.

0.6 Pass French Trail.

1.1 Pass Tres Sendas Trail.

1.6 Cross paved road (to the Chabot Space and Science Center). Pass just below the center.

1.7 Cross another road to continue on West Ridge Trail.

2.0 Redwood Bowl Picnic Area; pass Graham Trail.

2.1 Pass Redwood Peak and Madrone trail turnoffs.

2.6 Turn left on **Fern Trail**.

3.0 Turn left on **French Trail**. Veer left immediately to stay on French Trail.

3.5 Pass Mill Trail.

4.1 Pass Madrone Trail.

4.3 Cross Star Flower Trail.

4.5 Pass Redwood Trail.

5.0 Turn right on **Tres Sendas Trail**, signed also To French Trail.

5.1 Turn left on **French Trail**.

5.7 Turn right on **West Ridge Trail**.

You begin on the West Ridge Trail, a smooth, wide fire road that runs through oak, bay laurel, and an occasional stand of redwoods. Large madrones curve over the trail, and huckleberry adds its graceful foliage. The spicy scent of currants fills the air in winter. Views across the canyon of the East Bay hills and beyond to Mount Diablo provide immediate reward. An occasional short, steep uphill interrupts gentle ups and downs as the trail hugs the ridge. You cross beneath the large glass windows and aluminum siding of the impressive Chabot Space and Science Center, where you have westward views across the bay to the peninsula.

The trail enters a redwood forest and soon passes Redwood Bowl, an open glen with picnic tables. Here the West Ridge Trail leaves the redwoods and enters a grove of tall eucalyptus. You'll have great views of Contra Costa County's rolling hills to the east as you descend along the ridgeline on this exposed, sandstone trail. Redwood forest lies to the left of the ridge and dry chaparral covers the slopes to the right.

Once you join the Fern Trail you'll be on singletrack trails for nearly the rest of the route. The Fern Trail descends gradually, first through oak, bay laurel, toyon, and hemlock, and then quickly drops into a forest of redwoods, hazelnut, and ferns. Switchbacks make for an easy descent on the smooth dirt trail.

Your route up the length of densely forested Redwood Canyon follows the French Trail, a rollercoaster of steep ascents and descents. You climb up and down the hillside, crossing numerous paths, and occasionally following a seasonal creekbed. Tall redwoods let only a sprinkle of sunlight through their foliage, creating a cool haven in hot weather. In winter and spring, the lush understory is alive with growth—vibrant green hazelnut leaves, purple hound's tongue blossoms, and tiny star flowers.

The French Trail briefly joins the Tres Sendas Trail and then branches left to climb out of the redwood canyon. Oak and bay laurel take over the forest and sunlight cascades through the trees in delicate patterns. As you gain elevation the terrain becomes increasingly drier and the air warmer, and madrones appear in the forest. Watch for roots and rocks in the trail and poison oak along the sides. You may see False Solomon's seal, iris, and fairy bells here. Flat sections break the climb back to West Ridge, which becomes increasingly steep as you near the ridge. Look to the right for views of East Ridge across the canyon.

You rejoin the West Ridge Trail and retrace your steps for just over half a mile back to the trailhead.

Alternate Routes For a longer route, continue on the West Ridge Trail past the Fern Trail to the Chown Trail. Descend to the French Trail and follow it up the canyon, for a total run of about 7.5 miles.

If you're looking for something shorter, descend the Madrone Trail to the French Trail for a 4.5-mile loop. And if that isn't short enough, descend the very steep Tres Sendas Trail and climb back to West Ridge on the French Trail—about 2.75 miles total.

Trail Notes
- Singletrack and fire trails
- Some rock and root obstacles on the French Trail
- Dogs off leash on this route; must be leashed on Stream and Bridle trails
- No bikes on singletrack trails (Fern and French trails on this route)
- Horses allowed, except on Fern Trail during seasonal closures (usually through rainy season into early spring)
- Toilet and water at trailhead; water at Redwood Bowl Picnic Area (2.0 miles)
- No fees
- Heavily used park, but trails aren't crowded

 See suggestions in West Ridge Loop (Run 24).

ANTHONY CHABOT REGIONAL PARK

Anthony Chabot Regional Park covers almost 5,000 acres in the hills above Oakland and San Leandro. Despite the expanse, relatively few trails travel the park's open grasslands and sparse forests. The narrow lowland known as Grass Valley bisects the park lengthwise, and Grass Valley Creek runs through its center (dammed at the south end to form Lake Chabot). Two ridges rise gently on either side.

Non-native eucalyptus trees are ubiquitous in Chabot, but offer welcome shade in the exposed grasslands (increasingly taken over by coyote bush) that cover most of the park. You'll also find stands of redwoods, creekbeds surrounded by lush vegetation, and fragrant oak-and-bay woodlands.

At the southern reaches of the park, Lake Chabot is popular with families and locals as a picnic and boating destination. However, many areas of the park are seldom-visited. With few people on these trails, you have a good chance of glimpsing a fox or a coyote, and an even better chance of seeing hawks, rabbits, and deer.

Chabot Regional Park trailheads leave from the Equestrian Center and Grass Valley Staging Area on Skyline Boulevard, and the MacDonald, Bort Meadow, and Marciel Gate staging areas on Redwood Road. The East Bay Skyline National Recreation Trail and the Bay Area Ridge Trail run through Chabot, linking the park to Redwood Regional Park to the north and Cull Canyon Regional Recreation Area to the south.

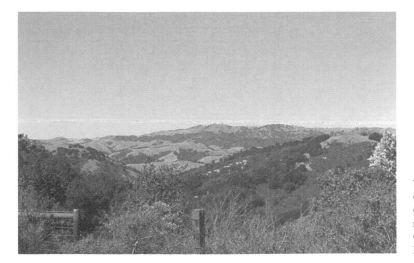

View of Contra Costa County Hills from Anthony Chabot Regional Park

What You'll Find Trails in Chabot Regional Park are open to dogs, bikes, horses, hikers, and runners, with certain restrictions. Bikes are allowed only on fire roads. Horses are allowed on most all trails, although singletracks are often off limits for equestrians in the rainy season. Toilets and water are available in certain locations—check individual runs for specifics.

26

GOLDENROD LOOP

From Chabot's exposed west ridge you drop into a secluded creek-side ravine, then emerge into a broad valley, and return to the ridge on a steep singletrack. Much of this route is exposed and can be hot in summer and muddy in winter.

Distance	8.5 miles
Time	1-2.25 hours
Type	loop
High Point/Low Point	1062'/245'
Difficulty	moderate
Use	light
Maps	EBRPD map
Area Management	East Bay Regional Park District

From Hwy. 13 in Oakland, take the Redwood Rd. exit and head east on Redwood Rd. Turn right on Skyline Blvd. and follow it 2.2 miles to the Equestrian Center. Turn left into the center and park in the dirt lot on your immediate left. **Trailhead Access**

Route Directions	Begin on unsigned singletrack across paved entrance road from parking lot.

Route Directions

Begin on unsigned singletrack across paved entrance road from parking lot.

0.1 Turn right on **Goldenrod Trail**.

0.4 Veer left on lower fork of Goldenrod Trail.

1.9 Pass Jackson Grade; upper fork of Goldenrod Trail rejoins your trail.

2.0 Pass Grass Valley Staging Area.

3.0 Turn left, signed TO COLUMBINE TRAIL.

3.3 Turn left on **Cascade Trail**.

4.3 Continue straight at stone bridge on **Brandon Trail**.

5.5 Pass Horseshoe Trail.

5.8 Unsigned fork; stay straight on the left (west) side of the meadow (right fork goes to Grass Valley Trail and Bort Meadow Staging Area).

6.2 Cross Bort Meadow to east side.

6.3 Follow gravel road right to meet **Grass Valley Trail**. Turn left, signed TO RANCH TRAIL, and go through metal cattle gate.

7.0 Curve left on **Ranch Trail** and go through cattle gate.

7.1 Turn left on **Goldenrod Trail**.

7.4 Pass Buckeye Trail.

8.3 Trail joins paved road at large water tank. Veer left to stay on Goldenrod Trail; paved road continues straight.

About the Trail

Begin this route on a narrow trail that leaves the parking lot and heads south along Skyline Blvd. beneath pine trees. You quickly join the Goldenrod Trail, a wide trail that follows the exposed ridgetop. High grasses, French broom, coyote bush, mugwort, and blackberry border the trail, and you have great views across Grass Valley to the rolling hills beyond. At a fork in the trail, take the lower path; on gentle descents and level stretches, the trail traces the contours of the hillside. Eucalyptus provide somewhat more shade than on the upper fork.

The upper and lower forks converge at Jackson Grade, which descends into the valley, and you continue on the Goldenrod Trail past the Grass Valley Staging Area and several homes that border the park.

The ridgeline begins a gentle downhill slope and you turn left and head into Grass Valley, past eucalyptus and abundant French broom. You reach the Cascade Trail, the gem of this route, a narrow singletrack that follows the ravine of Grass Valley Creek. Big-leaf maple, oak, and bay laurel shade the path. Sticky monkeyflower, cur-

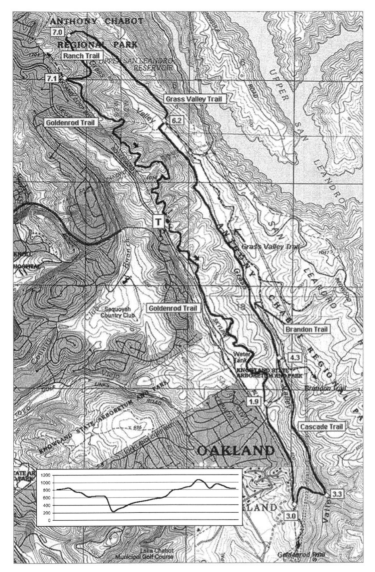

GOLDENROD LOOP

rants, and honeysuckle vines grow alongside, and by late spring, mugwort, cow parsnip, and bee plant crowd the trail. Ubiquitous poison oak reaches into the trail at every opportunity. (With a lot of care you can avoid it, but if you're particularly sensitive, avoid the trail completely during spring.)

The Cascade Trail ends at a stone bridge, and the Grass Valley and Brandon trails begin parallel routes along opposite sides of the willow-lined creek. The Grass Valley Trail passes through a eucalyptus grove to emerge on a wide, exposed trail, often in the company of grazing cows. The Brandon Trail is a cooler route, initially under the shade of redwoods and big-leaf maple. Poison oak, blackberry, coffeeberry, and cow parsnip crowd the trailside, and wild cucumber climbs the tree trunks. The trails converge again at Bort Meadow, a large grassy expanse at the head of Grass Valley, surrounded by eucalyptus and bay.

Cross the meadow to the gravel turnaround and toilets on the east side. Follow the gravel path briefly to the left-branching Grass Valley Trail (TO RANCH TRAIL). The narrow trail winds through high grasses and wild radish, and then crosses a small creekbed and heads up the ridge on exposed switchbacks. The loose-dirt trail is hot and dry in summer, but bay laurel and oak trees shade your way as the incline steepens.

Back on the ridgetop Goldenrod Trail, you have views into Grass Valley and beyond. The wide trail rolls up and down past dry hillsides of lupine, sticky monkeyflower, and sagebrush, and winds in and out of oak- and bay-shaded gullies. You go around a water tank and rejoin the trail on the far side, and then shortly return to the trailhead.

Alternate Routes For a shorter route—or if you're sensitive to poison oak—take Jackson Grade instead of the Cascade Trail. Turn left on Jackson Grade from the Goldenrod Trail and descend to the stone bridge, where you turn left on the Brandon Trail.

Trail Notes • Fire and singletrack trails
• Loose dirt on steep Ranch Trail; parts of Ranch and Cascade trails are narrow; abundant poison oak on Cascade Trail; sticky mud on Grass Valley Trail.
• Dogs off leash, under voice control
• Bikes allowed on Goldenrod, Grass Valley, and Brandon trails on this route
• Horses allowed on all trails on this route
• Restrooms and water at trailhead in stable building
• Toilets and water at Bort Meadow
• No fees

- You'll see only an occasional hiker or runner in Chabot Regional Park. Mountain bikers and equestrians also use the trails, but overall the park is lightly used.
- Don't be alarmed when you hear the sound of shots ringing through the woods. The Marksmanship Range is open Wednesday through Friday, from 10 AM to 5 PM and weekends from 9 AM to 5 PM.

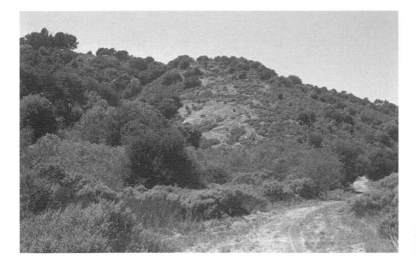

Grass Valley Trail, looking toward Ranch Trail

27

BORT MEADOW LOOP

This run traverses the floor of wide, picturesque Grass Valley, climbs to the east ridge of the park for views of the Contra Costa County hills, and descends back into the valley on wide, mostly exposed trails.

Distance	7.2 miles
Time	1–1.75 hours
Type	semi-loop
High Point/Low Point	929′/498′
Difficulty	moderate
Use	light
Maps	EBRPD map at trailhead
Area Management	East Bay Regional Park District

Trailhead Access From Hwy. 13 in Oakland, take the Redwood Rd. exit. Head east on Redwood Rd. Cross Skyline Blvd. and continue on Redwood Rd. Where Pinehurst Rd. veers left, stay right on Redwood Rd. and continue another 2 miles to Bort Meadow Staging Area (also called Big Trees).

Route Directions Follow paved road from south end of parking area.
Turn left on **Grass Valley Trail** (part of the Bay Area Ridge Trail and the East Bay Skyline National Recreation Trail).
1.0 Pass Redtail Trail.
1.5 Turn left on **Brandon Trail**, also signed LAKE CHABOT BICYCLE LOOP.
1.7 Pass Cottontail Trail.
2.1 Turn right on **Escondido Trail**.
3.6 Turn left on **Brandon Trail**.
4.1 Turn right on spur trail signed TO REDTAIL TRAIL.
4.2 Turn left on **Redtail Trail**.

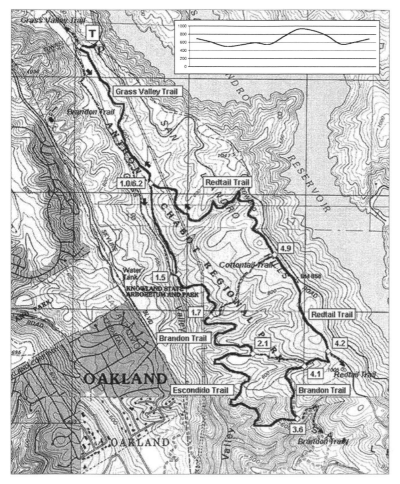

BORT MEADOW LOOP

4.3 Cross Marciel Rd. and continue on Redtail Trail.
4.8 Marciel Gate parking area; cross parking lot to continue on
  Redtail Trail.
4.9 Pass Cottontail Trail.
6.2 Turn right on **Grass Valley Trail.**

You begin on the level Grass Valley Trail, through open, cow-grazed   **About the**
pastures. Coyote bush and scrub oak dot grassy slopes that border the   **Trail**
trail to the east, and the densely forested slopes of the west ridge rise
across the valley. The valley narrows as you near the Brandon Trail,

and eucalyptus trees, interspersed with redwood and big-leaf maple, shade the trail.

You turn right at the stone bridge on the Brandon Trail. Eucalyptus trees still provide sparse shade along the wide trail. Coyote bush, ferns, blackberry, wild cucumber, gooseberry, and poison oak cover the hillside, despite the abundance of invasive French broom and pampas grass.

High grasses on the Escondido Trail indicate that it is not a well-traveled route. After a gentle downgrade, the trail levels in a ravine, under a dense cover of oaks and eucalyptus. You climb out of the ravine and rejoin the Brandon Trail, where you'll have views west of Oakland and San Leandro and across the bay to San Francisco.

Bay laurel, coffeeberry, coyote bush, grasses, and sticky monkeyflower line the smooth and level Brandon Trail. Where the trail curves to the left around a gully, you branch right on a spur to the Redtail Trail. Climb steeply to the ridgetop on the rutted, grassy trail. Views of the rolling East Bay hills greet you: upper San Leandro Reservoir is hidden in a deep valley; undulating ridges rise beyond it and Mt. Diablo crests in the distance.

These views accompany you on the singletrack Redtail Trail along the exposed ridgeline. In spring, low-lying sun cups brighten the trail. Past the Cottontail Trail, your route widens, winds through open hills, and dips into lush creek ravines crowded with bay laurel, big-leaf maple, cow parsnip, ferns, and morning glory.

Beyond a cattle gate, you descend into Grass Valley, first gradually, then more steeply. Across the valley you see the Goldenrod Trail (Run 26) on the west ridge; to the north, the McDonald Trail, part of the Bay Area Ridge Trail, traverses the east ridge. When you reach the floor of Grass Valley, turn right and follow the first mile of your route to return to the trailhead.

Alternate Routes The Brandon Trail runs through Grass Valley, parallel to the Grass Valley Trail, on the other side of the creek. It is a useful alternative during the rainy season because it is somewhat less muddy than the Grass Valley Trail.

To begin on the Brandon Trail, instead of turning left immediately at the bottom of the paved road from the trailhead, continue straight on the wide gravel path to the open meadow just ahead, and then turn left on the wide dirt Brandon Trail. At the stone bridge

(1.5 miles), turn left again, staying on the Brandon Trail, and follow the route description from there.

For a shorter loop (6.1 miles), skip the Escondido Trail and stay on the Brandon Trail to the Redtail Trail. The views from the Redtail Trail are one of the highlights of this run, so don't miss that part of the route!

- Fire trails with one singletrack section on Redtail Trail
- Mostly smooth trails, although rutted in summer and fall from dry mud and hoof prints; Escondido Trail sometimes overgrown; Grass Valley Trail exposed and hot during summer; sticky mud during the rainy season, worsened by cows
- Dogs off leash, under voice control
- Bikes allowed on all trails on this route
- Horses allowed on all trails on this route
- Toilets, water at Bort Meadow, 0.25 mile north of the trailhead
- No fees
- You'll see only an occasional hiker or runner in Chabot Regional Park. Mountain bikers and equestrians also use the trails, but overall the park is lightly used.
- Don't be alarmed when you hear the sound of shots ringing through the woods. The Marksmanship Range is open Wednesday through Friday, from 10 AM to 5 PM and weekends from 9 AM to 5 PM.

The sticky mud that plagues many East Bay trails during the rainy season is a result of soil composition. Most soils contain a mixture of clay, sand, silt, and other organic matter; soils that contain a high percentage of clay particles, such as those in the East Bay, are called clay soils. The fine clay particles bind together by the process of cohesion. When wet, they coalesce into sticky masses that cling to the bottoms of your shoes. In summer, clay soils become jigsaw puzzles of dry earth. As the sun bakes the dirt, the clumps of soil harden and split apart, forming deep fissures that resemble miniature fault lines.

BRIONES REGIONAL PARK

Once the heart of Contra Costa ranchland, the rolling grassy hills of Briones Regional Park are now a 5,756-acre natural refuge from the sprawling towns of Orinda, Lafayette, and Walnut Creek. Creeks surge through broad valleys in the rainy season and reduce to a meager trickle in the hot summer months. Rollercoaster ridges rise from these lowlands, and offer 360-degree views of Contra Costa County —the Sacramento River delta flows toward the bay from the Sierra

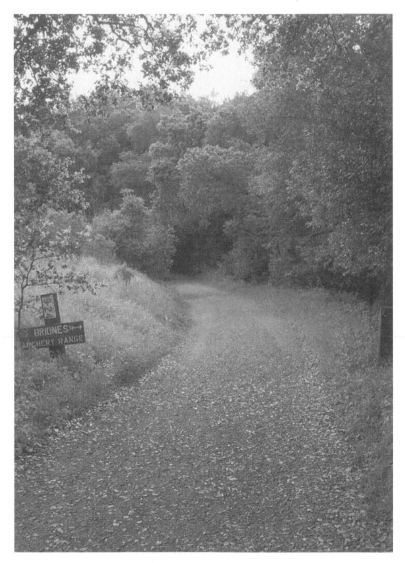

Oak trees shade
the Homestead
Valley Trail

Nevada, Mt. Diablo rises beyond suburban communities to the east, and San Pablo Ridge stands between the coast and these valleys.

Like many parts of the East Bay, this was ranchland in the 19th and early 20th centuries. Cattle grazing played an important role in shaping the appearance of the landscape by introducing European annual grasses that cover the hills. Although now part of the EBRPD, the land is still heavily grazed, and if not for the cows, these grasses could become major fire hazards. The cows reduce the brush that would take over the grasslands, but they also encourage the growth of yellow star thistle, an invasive plant you'll see growing on these hillsides. The large patties along the trail are also signs of the cows' presence.

Briones is best enjoyed in late spring and fall. The broad fire trails that run up and down the hills are muddy in winter and during early spring, and summers are HOT. But autumn in Briones is enchanting—all that remains of the summer's heat are golden grasses on the open hillsides and baked-earth trails. Big-leaf maples turn brilliant colors in wooded creek ravines. By late fall, Briones' freshwater ponds fill with water, and you will hear the sounds of frogs croaking as you pass by.

The two main trailheads for Briones Regional Park are the Alhambra Valley Staging Area, off Reliez Valley Road near Martinez, and the Bear Creek Road Staging Area near Orinda and Lafayette. The featured runs begin from Bear Creek.

What You'll Find

Trails in Briones Regional Park are open to dogs, bikes, horses, hikers, and runners, with certain restrictions. Bikes are allowed only on fire roads. The Abrigo Valley Trail has been resurfaced as far as the group camps (about 1.4 miles), making it a good route for jogging strollers. Toilets and water are available at the Bear Creek trailhead and the Wee-Ta Chi and Maud Whalen trail camps (on the Abrigo Valley Trail at the junctions with the Santos and Mott Peak trails). The park charges a $4 entrance fee and $1 dog fee when the kiosk is staffed.

28

BRIONES CREST LOOP

This exposed route climbs to the ridgeline along an offshoot of Bear Creek and loops around three valleys. On stiff ups and downs you'll skirt Mott and Briones peaks and descend beside another creekbed.

Distance	8 miles
Time	1-2 hours
Type	loop
High Point/Low Point	1428´/704´
Difficulty	moderate
Use	light
Maps	EBRPD map at trailhead
Area Management	East Bay Regional Park District

Trailhead Access Take the Orinda exit from Hwy. 24 and turn north on Camino Pablo. Go 2.2 miles to Bear Creek Rd. Turn right and continue 4.5 miles to the Bear Creek Road Staging Area. Turn right and continue 0.3 mile to the entrance kiosk. Park in the far left parking area.

Route Directions Begin on paved road from easternmost parking area. Follow signs to Old Briones Rd. and Homestead Valley trails.

0.2 Veer right on **Homestead Valley Trail** at junction with Old Briones Rd.

0.6 Turn right on Homestead Valley Trail at junction with Crescent Ridge Trail.

0.7 Pass Bear Creek Trail.

1.8 Turn left on **Briones Crest Trail.**

2.3 Pass Crescent Ridge Trail.

2.4 Pass No Name Trail.

2.7 Turn left on **Briones Crest Trail** at junction with Table Mountain Trail.

3.2 Pass Valley Trail.

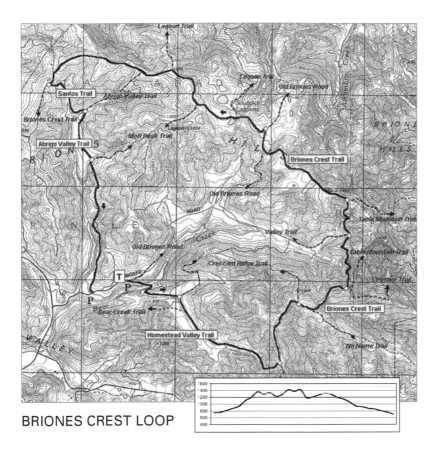

BRIONES CREST LOOP

3.5 Turn left on **Briones Crest Trail** at second junction with Table Mountain Trail.

4.4 Turn left on Briones Crest Trail at junction with Old Briones Rd.

4.6 Pass Lagoon Trail.

4.9 Pass Mott Peak Trail.

5.3 Pass Lagoon Trail again.

5.5 Pass Abrigo Valley Trail.

6.3 Turn left on **Santos Trail.**

6.7 Turn right on **Abrigo Valley Trail.**

7.1 Turn right on Abrigo Valley Trail at junction with Mott Peak Trail.

About the Trail From the easternmost parking lot (on your right when you drive in), you briefly follow a paved road toward Old Briones Road and Homestead Valley trails. Look to the left at the hills that rise steeply from the valley; you'll often see raptors soaring above them. Coyote bush lines the road, in full, fuzzy bloom in fall.

Shortly you descend into the ravine of Bear Creek on the wide, gravel Homestead Valley Trail. Bay laurel's strong fragrance permeates the air. In fall, big-leaf maple, poison oak, and blackberry turn muted reds and golds. You climb out of the ravine and emerge in broad Homestead Valley. Grassy hills ripple upward from the valley floor, spotted with oak and bay. Willows grow in dense stands along the creek.

The trail continues level through the valley. It is muddy in the rainy season and rutted by cow hooves in summer. Invasive yellow star thistle thrives in soil disturbed by grazing cows and grows rampantly in valleys and on grassy hillsides. The valley narrows and the trail enters a fold in the hills to begin a gentle climb. Oak and bay laurel branches high above the trail offer light shade. The ascent steepens as you near the Briones Crest Trail.

Graceful old oaks line the Briones Crest Trail, shading it in parts. The wide, smooth trail rolls along the ridgeline with some steep ups and downs. You have views to the left into Briones and beyond to San Pablo Ridge, and to the right, past the hills surrounding Lafayette Reservoir to Mt. Diablo.

You soon descend from the ridge into a shady ravine, its hillsides covered with oak and bay laurel. A gradual ascent up an open hillside becomes steeper and shaded as you near the ridgeline again. Gravel and dirt overlay the sandstone trail. Once at the ridgetop you climb again briefly, passing Briones Peak, the highest point in the park at 1483 feet.

You can see the wide, graveled trail ahead of you as it winds around oak-topped knolls. You descend gently, with views northeast toward Martinez and the delta, west into the valleys of Briones and to San Pablo Ridge. Mott Peak (1424´) tops the barren hills ahead of you. You soon pass two freshwater ponds—a rare sight in the Bay Area hills—surrounded by cattails and reeds, and climb gradually around the east side of Mott Peak. The trail undulates over rippled hills and grasses rustle in the breeze on these high ridges.

You turn left on the Santos Trail and descend steeply into Abrigo Valley. The trail levels next to a willow-lined creek in the valley, and buckeyes grow on the hillside—their sturdy bare branches hung with round chestnuts in fall and winter, and in spring, adorned with white flower stalks.

You finish this route on the level Abrigo Valley Trail; the hard-packed gravel surface ameliorates muddy conditions in wet weather. The dense cover of oak and bay laurel trees on the hillside across the creek is interspersed with madrones, identified by their red trunks even from this distance.

You can easily create a longer or a shorter route with the many trails that traverse Briones. One option is to follow Old Briones Road to the Briones Crest Trail, and then turn left on the Crest Trail and follow the rest of the featured route (5.2 miles). **Alternate Routes**

Trail Notes

- Fire trails
- Wide, smooth trails; excessively muddy in the rainy season
- Dogs off leash, under voice control; $1 dog fee
- Bikes allowed on all trails on this route
- Horses allowed
- Toilet and water at trailhead; toilets on Abrigo Valley Trail (at junctions with Santos and Mott Peak trails)
- $4/day fee when kiosk is staffed (rarely)
- The first 1.4 miles of the Abrigo Valley Trail is a good route for jogging strollers.
- The charred grasslands you may see in late summer and fall are most likely the result of controlled burns conducted by the park district.

COYOTE HILLS REGIONAL PARK

A small oasis of wildlife and Native American history tucked on the outskirts Fremont, Coyote Hills is an unexpected treasure. These protected hills and marshlands feel surprisingly remote from the densely populated and industrialized surrounding area.

You'll find three predominant landscapes at Coyote Hills: bay, marshlands, and grasslands. East of the visitor center, across Patterson Ranch Road, wide, smooth dirt trails lined by high cattails crisscross the marshlands. Behind the visitor center, Glider and Red hills rise between the marshland and the bay. Wide dirt trails run the length of the hills and provide short, steep climbs. These high points provide great views of the area—west across the bay to the Santa Cruz Mountains, and east beyond the marshlands to the Diablo Range.

To experience the rich shoreline environment at Coyote Hills, take the 3.5-mile paved loop on the Bayview Trail around the grassy knobs of Coyote and Red hills. The Pelican Trail extends north of the Bayview Trail, an unpaved singletrack that connects to the paved Alameda Creek Trail. Apay Way, also unpaved, runs south from the Bayview Trail and leads to the Don Edwards San Francisco National Wildlife Refuge (after crossing a pedestrian overpass above Highway 84).

Once you understand the lay of the land at Coyote Hills, the park is small enough to easily explore on your own, with or without a map. The featured route takes you through the marshlands, along the bayshore, and up and down the grassy hills—it includes a few good climbs, easy running on flat, smooth trails, and a wilder singletrack.

What You'll Find   Coyote Hills Regional Park is open to dogs, bikes, and horses. Check the featured route for individual trail rules. The park is open from 8 AM to 8 PM April to October, and 8 AM to 6 PM November to March. There is a $2 entrance fee on weekends and holidays and a $1 dog fee. The visitor center, open Thursday through Sunday, 9:30 AM to 5 PM, has exhibits on the park's wildlife and Native American history. Restrooms and water are at the visitor center.

29

COYOTE HILLS ROUNDABOUT

This exposed loop combines short, steep climbs on the bayside hills with long, flat stretches at bay level. You'll enjoy views east of the marshlands and Mission Peak, and west across the bay to the northern ridge of the Santa Cruz Mountains. Look for herons, egrets, and ducks in the marshes, and rabbits and muskrats along the trails. You'll be on pavement for about half a mile.

Distance	4.5 miles
Time	0.5–1.25 hours
Type	loop
High Point/Low Point	263´/3´
Difficulty	moderate
Use	moderate
Maps	EBRPD map at visitor center
Area Management	EBRPD

Take Hwy. 880 to the Decoto Rd./Hwy. 84 exit in Fremont. Head west on Hwy. 84 to the Thornton Ave./Paseo Padre Pkwy. exit. Go north on Paseo Padre for less than a mile and turn left on Patterson Ranch Rd. Continue to the park entrance.

**Trailhead
Access**

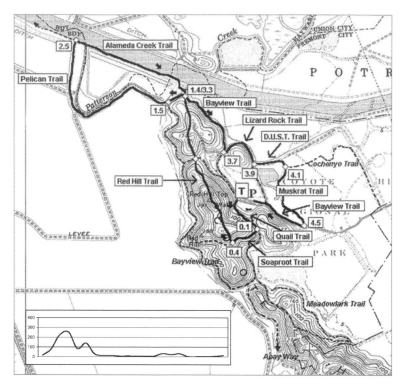

COYOTE HILLS ROUNDABOUT

Route Directions

Begin just north of the visitor center on the **Quail Trail** (signed SOAPROOT TRAIL).

0.1 Turn right sharply on **Soaproot Trail**.

0.4 Turn right on **Red Hill Trail**.

1.4 Turn left on **Bayview Trail**.

1.5 Turn right on unsigned **Pelican Trail**.

2.5 Turn right on **Alameda Creek Trail**.

3.3 Turn right on **Bayview Trail**.

3.7 Turn left on **Lizard Rock Trail**.

3.9 Turn left on **D.U.S.T. Trail**.

4.1 Turn right on **Muskrat Trail**.

4.2 Continue straight where the Chochenyo Trail branches left.

4.3 Continue straight where the Muskrat Trail branches left.

4.5 Turn right to return along the **Bayview Trail** to the visitor center.

This route begins behind the visitor center to the north. On the EBRPD map, the trail appears to be the Quail Trail, but a signpost designates this wide, graveled road the Soaproot Trail. At the crest of a small rise, you turn onto a smooth dirt path that continues up the hill. Dairy Glen Picnic Area is below you; the paved Bayview Trail skirts the picnic tables on its way to the bay shore.

You climb Glider Hill on a short but steep ascent and quickly descend the other side, where you can see ahead to the red-dirt trail that climbs Red Hill. Fennel and mustard grow on these grassy hills and raptors swoop above them. Take in the views both east and west: Look down on the rich tapestry of the marshlands, where the cattails and tules change from green to golden with the seasons. The hills beyond rise east of the flat bay plain, and the industry of Fremont is barely noticeable from this vantage. To the west you have views of the salt marshes, the bay, and the Santa Cruz Mountains beyond.

You pass the Nike Trail and endure another abrupt up and down on the Red Hill Trail before turning left on the paved Bayview Trail. Just beyond, look for the Pelican Trail, marked with a hiker sign. This unkempt trail becomes an overgrown singletrack with some of the best scenery and wildlife in Coyote Hills. The trail traces a small spit of land between salt ponds and marshland. Pickleweed in the marsh turns brilliant magenta in fall; evaporation in the salt ponds turns the water from greenish to light pink, influenced by algae and brine shrimp. You brush through high grasses until the trail broadens and turns inland. As you near the Alameda Creek Trail, look for egrets and herons in the salt ponds on your left.

Back on the Bayview Trail, you round Red Hill on its eastern side, and in less than half a mile you turn on the dirt Lizard Rock Trail. Follow this wide level trail through grasslands toward the marsh. On the D.U.S.T. Trails, you are surrounded by the marsh. Ducks and other water birds congregate in the water, and high cattails and tules rise on either side, obscuring all but the rippled ridges of the Diablo Range and the sky. You feel miles away from the freeway and industrial parks. Wind through the marsh on these short trails and then leave it via a wooden pathway over the waters and return to the visitor center.

For views south toward the Dumbarton Bridge and east into the marsh, the Meadowlark Trail makes a good route, combining a paved hill trail and a flat dirt trail along the marsh. Tackle this 2.3-mile loop on its own or combine it with other trails for a longer run.

Trail Notes
- Singletrack, wide, and paved trails
- Generally smooth; Pelican Trail overgrown in sections; Red Hill Trail steep in sections; may be bad mud patches on Muskrat Trail
- Dogs must be leashed; not allowed in wetland, marsh, or visitor center area; dog fee
- Bikes allowed on paved Bayview Trail, and on Red Hill and Soaproot trails on this route.
- Horses allowed on paved Bayview Trail, and on Red Hill, Quail, and Soaproot trails on this route.
- Toilet and water at visitor center

Nature Notes

The knob-like mounds of Red Hill are named for the rust-colored Franciscan chert that underlies Coyote Hills. Chert is composed of one-celled marine animals called radiolarians that settled on the ocean floor millions of years ago; its red color results from iron deposits that later oxidized with exposure to the air. Chert is a strong rock and highly resistant to erosion, which is why the rounded protusions of Red Hill have kept their shape while the surrounding land has been worn away to form a level bay plain.

SUNOL REGIONAL WILDERNESS

In the vast 6,858 acres of Sunol Regional Wilderness it's easy to imagine you are much farther from the busy Bay Area than you really are. High peaks crown Sunol's oak-studded hillsides, and rocky outcroppings form an impressive landscape. Alameda Creek, the largest stream in Alameda County, courses along the southern border of the park through a dramatic rockbound canyon—Little Yosemite Gorge. The Ohlone Regional Wilderness Trail (Run 30) crosses Sunol Regional Wilderness on its 28-mile route from Mission Peak Regional Preserve to Del Valle Regional Park. To the east and west, San Francisco Water Department land abuts the park, with Calaveras Reservoir in prominent view from the park's high points.

Ranches occupied this land before the EBRPD purchased it, and cattle still graze on the hillsides and leave large patties along the trails. Sunol can get very hot in summer; run these trails in early morning, or better yet, in spring, fall, or winter. In spring, wildflowers blanket the hillsides, including poppies, lupine, blue dicks, and goldfields. In chilly fall, big-leaf maple, sycamores, alders, and willows lose their golden leaves.

What You'll Find

Sunol Regional Wilderness is open from 7 AM to dusk year round, unless otherwise posted. There is a $4 parking fee and a $1 dog fee.

Dogs must be on leash on the Indian Joe Nature Trail and on Camp Ohlone Road. They can be off-leash and under voice control on other trails, but be sure your dog really *is* under control, since Sunol is a popular equestrian park. Bikes and horses are allowed on fire roads, and horses are also allowed on the singletrack Ohlone Wilderness Trail through Sunol. Several singletrack trails are for foot traffic only. Check individual runs for specifics on trail-use regulations.

Beyond Sunol's boundaries, the Ohlone Wilderness Trail crosses San Francisco Water Department land; you must have a permit if you continue on the trail outside of the park. You can purchase one for $2 at the Sunol entrance kiosk.

Toilets are located in the main parking lot and at the junction of Cerro Este and Camp Ohlone roads. Water is available at the main entrance's far parking lot. The visitor center at the main entrance is a good place to find out more about Sunol's trails and natural history.

Sunol's main trailhead, on Geary Road near the visitor center, is the best access point for most trails. Another trailhead on Welch

Creek Road is a good starting point for a trip to Maguire Peaks (pick up a permit at the Geary Road visitor center in order to park on Welch Creek Road; if you are a Regional Parks Foundation member, just leave your card on the dashboard).

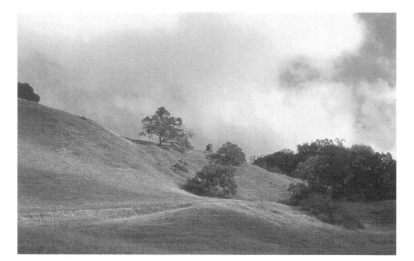

Sunol's
golden hills

30

OHLONE WILDERNESS TRAIL LOOP

This exposed loop crosses steep hillsides and follows creekbeds on singletrack and wide trails, with a detour into the exceptional Little Yosemite Gorge. Weathered rock outcroppings and massive valley and coast live oaks punctuate the grasslands. Wildflowers carpet the hills in spring and deciduous maples and sycamores color the ground in fall.

Distance	6.2 miles
Time	0.75–1.5 hours
Type	semi-loop
High Point/Low Point	1441′/397′
Difficulty	moderate
Use	light
Maps	EBRPD map at trailhead and visitor center
Area Management	East Bay Regional Park District

Trailhead Access

From I-680, exit at Calaveras Rd./Hwy. 84. Turn south on Calaveras Rd. After 4.2 miles, turn left on Geary Rd. at small brown regional park sign. Continue 1.7 miles to parking lot and visitor center.

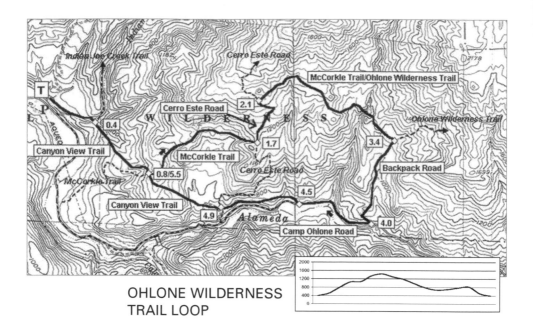

OHLONE WILDERNESS TRAIL LOOP

Route Directions Begin at trailhead next to toilets. Cross wooden bridge.
Turn right on **Canyon View Trail**, also Indian Joe Nature Trail.

0.2 Turn left on Canyon View Trail.

0.4 Veer right on Canyon View Trail; Indian Joe Creek Trail veers left.

0.8 Turn left on **McCorkle Trail**.

1.7 Turn left on **Cerro Este Rd.**

2.1 Turn right on **McCorkle Trail/Ohlone Wilderness Trail.**

3.4 Go straight on **Backpack Rd.**, faintly signed TO CANYON VIEW; Ohlone Wilderness Trail goes left.

4.0 Turn right on **Camp Ohlone Rd.**

4.3 Pass W Tree Rock Scramble.

4.5 Veer right on **Canyon View Trail.**

4.9 Turn right on Cerro Este Rd. to join Canyon View Trail. Make immediate left on Canyon View Trail.

5.5 Cross McCorkle Trail to continue on Canyon View and retrace steps to trailhead.

About the Trail This loop begins next to Alameda Creek, lined with big-leaf maple, sycamore, and willows. The wide trail is at first both the Indian Joe Nature Trail and the Canyon View Trail (also the Ohlone Wilderness

Trail). You cross a small tributary creek and head uphill on a short but stiff climb. Thickets of snowberry crowd the narrow, rolling trail along with abundant sagebrush and orange sticky monkeyflower. Rocks and oak tree roots clutter the path, and the trees provide little shade. Veer right to stay on the Canyon View Trail where the Indian Joe Trail goes left. On another stiff uphill, you pass through a cattle gate and climb wooden logs set across the trail to help prevent erosion.

You continue climbing, gently but steadily, dodging patties left by the cows that graze in pastures along the trail. The McCorkle Trail crosses the Canyon View Trail and you turn left on it; your return section of the Canyon View Trail goes straight. On the broad McCorkle Trail, you wind up the grassy hillside on a moderate but steady climb, taking in views of Sunol's high ridges, the rocky protuberance of Flag Hill, and then, as the trail swings to the left, Maguire Peaks.

The trail reaches a crest and veers right toward a chaparral-covered hillside. It becomes a narrow singletrack, lined by coyote bush, gooseberry, and sagebrush. After a level stretch the trail begins to climb, steeply at times. Oak and bay laurel trees and thickets of poison oak thrive along the creekbed that borders the trail.

On Cerro Este Road you continue climbing, now heading northeast on a wide trail. Massive oaks dot the hillsides, rising against vast open slopes and sky. You soon pick up the singletrack McCorkle Trail again and head further into Sunol's wilderness, following the Ohlone Wilderness Trail toward Del Valle. A small footpath heads left, but your route continues on the Ohlone Wilderness Trail. The singletrack cuts across rolling hillsides where enormous rocky outcroppings accompany solitary oaks. You cross many small creekbeds, often dry; big-leaf maple and bay laurel trees grow among dark, glossy boulders in larger streambeds.

Stay on the main trail, avoiding small paths that stray from it, especially on a steep hillside descent where logs hold eroding dirt in place. You have views of Calaveras Reservoir high beyond the deep gorge of Alameda Creek. After one last creek crossing, you leave the Ohlone Wilderness Trail and descend a wide, well-graded trail. You reach the broad canyon of Alameda Creek and turn right to follow its westward course. The wide, gravelly Camp Ohlone Road descends through oaks, and you look down on the rocky creekbed; in fall, deciduous sycamore and big-leaf maple trees and willow litter the dry watercourse.

Beyond a broad creek-side meadow you veer right on the Canyon View Trail. The narrow singletrack traverses the hillside above Camp Ohlone Road on a level course. (Keep to the main trail above the barbed wire fence.) After crossing a grassy, cow-patty-strewn field, you meet Cerro Este Road again.

To see the section of Alameda Creek called Little Yosemite, detour left on Cerro Este Road, a half-mile round trip. You meet Camp Ohlone Road and turn left to see the impressive gorge. (There is a toilet at Cerro Este and Camp Ohlone roads.) Return to the Cerro Este/Canyon View junction.

After a short jog on the Cerro Este Trail, you continue on the Canyon View Trail as it hugs a high, open hillside. You cross the McCorkle Trail and then retrace your steps on the steep trail you began on.

Alternate Routes For an easier route to Little Yosemite Gorge, do a 2-mile out-and-back trip on Camp Ohlone Road. To reach the trailhead, drive past the visitor center and park in the far parking lot. The wide, picturesque trail follows Alameda Creek, lined with lofty trees. You can continue beyond the gorge for about another three-quarters of a mile on Camp Ohlone Road if you want to extend this route.

Trail Notes
- Singletrack and fire trails
- Steep climbs, roots, and rocks on Canyon View and McCorkle trails; steep descent on Canyon View Trail, may be slippery
- Dogs on leash on Indian Joe Nature Trail and Camp Ohlone Road; otherwise off-leash, under voice control
- Bikes allowed on Cerro Este, Backpack, and Camp Ohlone roads
- Horses allowed Cerro Este, Backpack, and Camp Ohlone roads and McCorkle Trail
- Toilets at trailhead and at junction of Cerro Este and Camp Ohlone roads (short detour off trail)
- No water at trailhead; drinking fountain at far parking lot (Camp Ohlone Road trailhead)

 You'll find a few food choices in the town of Sunol. The Sunol Grocery stocks the basics, but a steakhouse and a café provide more filling options. To reach Sunol, pass under I-680 on Calaveras Road and follow signs to town.

From the McCorkle Trail, you can see the Calaveras Reservoir, part of the San Francisco Water District Department. Built in 1925, this massive earth- and rock-fill dam holds 31.5 million gallons of water, fed by Sierra Nevada snow pack and by westward flowing streams on their way to the bay.

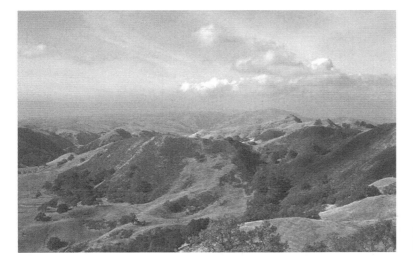

Looking towards
Maguire Peaks

31

CAVE ROCKS LOOP

On steep singletracks and fire trails, you'll pass a basalt rock outcrop, cross pastures and chaparral slopes, and absorb far-reaching views of Sunol's craggy ridges and billowing hills.

Distance	5.1 miles
Time	0.75–1.25 hours
Type	semi-loop
High Point/Low Point	1730′/397′
Difficulty	moderate
Use	light
Maps	EBRPD map at trailhead and visitor center
Area Management	East Bay Regional Park District

Trailhead Access
From I-680, exit at Calaveras Rd./Hwy. 84. Turn south on Calaveras Rd. After 4.2 miles, turn left on Geary Rd. at small brown regional park sign. Continue 1.7 miles to parking lot and visitor center.

Route Directions
Begin at trailhead next to toilets. Cross wooden bridge. Turn right on **Canyon View Trail**, also Indian Joe Nature Trail.
0.2 Turn left on Canyon View Trail.
0.4 Veer left on **Indian Joe Creek Trail**; Canyon View Trail veers right.
1.3 Pass Hayfield Rd.
1.6 Turn right on **Cave Rocks Rd.**
1.9 Pass Eagle View Rd.
2.0 Pass Eagle View Trail.
2.6 Turn right on **Cerro Este Rd.**
3.4 Turn right on **McCorkle Trail.**
4.3 Turn right on **Canyon View Trail.**
4.7 Meet **Indian Joe Creek Trail**; continue straight to retrace steps to trailhead.

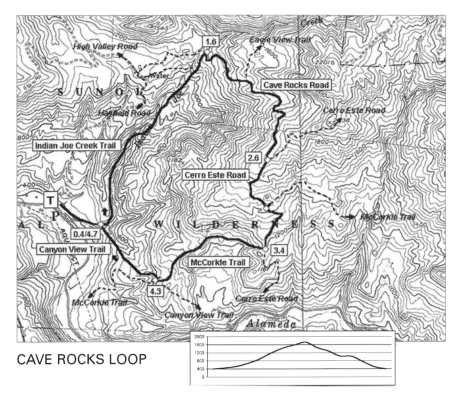

CAVE ROCKS LOOP

You begin this route by crossing the wooden bridge over Alameda Creek; big-leaf maple, sycamore, and willows line the wide streambed. You briefly follow the creek on a broad trail, here both the Indian Joe Nature Trail and the Canyon View Trail. Once across a small tributary creek, you veer uphill on a short but stiff climb. Roots from the sparse oak trees overhead push into the narrow trail, and snowberry bushes, sagebrush, and orange sticky monkeyflowers grow alongside. After a few short ups and downs, veer left on the Indian Joe Creek Trail where the Canyon View Trail, your return route, goes right.

Your singletrack trail follows Indian Joe Creek on a gentle but steady climb. Oak and big-leaf maple initially provide sparse shade; in fall, their leaves cover the ground in a colorful tapestry of golden and russet. The trail fords the creek, and blue dicks, buttercups, and other spring wildflowers bloom in a small grassy expanse. Occasional roots and a fallen bay laurel trunk create obstacles. The trail becomes rockier as you climb, and you pass the Hayfields Road junction. Take in

About the Trail

the view of the rolling hills and forested gulches that rise to the ridge on your right.

On a steep and gravelly section you pass Indian Joe Cave Rocks, a large basalt outcropping and a training spot for rock climbers. A few short switchbacks attempt to temper the grade as you make the final push to Cave Rocks Road.

You continue on a steady but gradual climb on wide Cave Rocks Road, accompanied by sweeping views to the east over high ridges and rolling hills, punctuated by majestic oaks. To your left, a lone rock on a ridgecrest pierces the skyline. Past left-branching Eagle View Road, your trail continues on a gentler grade. The singletrack Eagle View Trail veers left soon after, and you trudge up the last uphill stretch on Cave Rocks Road. Sunol's high peaks (2201′ and 2038′) rise from grassy slopes above you.

Turn right at a junction with Cerro Este Road and head down-hill on the broad trail. Solitary oaks rise from the rounded curves of the hillside and cows graze on the grassy slopes. Below you to the southwest, you can see the Calaveras reservoir in San Francisco Water Department land. You pass the left-branching McCorkle Trail and continue to find its right-hand extension.

The narrow McCorkle Trail initially descends steeply, and small, loose rocks may make the trail slippery. Thickets of poison oak grow beneath oak and bay laurel trees. The trail levels and emerges onto open chaparral slopes of coyote bush, gooseberry, and sagebrush. After a brief climb, you return to grassland and follow a broad trail gently downhill. Turn right on the singletrack Canyon View Trail and descend steeply in spots, watching for roots and rocks; wooden logs are laid across to help prevent erosion. You meet the Indian Joe Nature Trail and retrace your steps to the trailhead.

Alternate Routes If you're looking for a longer adventure, explore the remote Maguire Peaks Trail on the other side of Welch Creek Road. Turn left instead of right on Cave Rocks Road; then meet the High Valley Trail and cross Welch Creek Road to the Maguire Peaks Trail, which circles the rocky pinnacles of Maguire Peaks. From the junction of the Indian Joe Creek Trail and Cave Rocks Road and back, this adds about 8.1 miles to your run.

- Singletrack and fire trails
- Steep descent on McCorkle Trail, may be slippery; some roots and rocks, especially on Canyon View Trail; Cave Rocks Road may be muddy in wet weather; creek crossings in spring on Indian Joe Creek Trail; steep climb on Indian Joe
- Dogs on leash on Indian Joe Nature Trail and Camp Ohlone Road; otherwise off-leash, under voice control
- Bikes allowed on Cave Rocks and Cerro Este roads
- Horses allowed on Cave Rocks and Cerro Este roads and McCorkle Trail
- Toilets at trailhead
- No water at trailhead; drinking fountain at far parking lot (Camp Ohlone Road trailhead)

See the Ohlone Wilderness Trail Loop (Run 30) for suggestions.

EAST BAY MUNICIPAL UTILITY DISTRICT

East Bay Municipal Utilities District manages five reservoirs and more than 28,000 acres of land in the East Bay. Billions of gallons of water are pumped across the Central Valley from the Sierra Nevada and stored in these reservoirs to serve the Bay Area's water needs. The reservoirs and surrounding watershed lands supply Bay Area residents with recreational opportunities. Fishing, boating, and picnicking are popular activities at San Pablo, Chabot, and Lafayette reservoirs, and a regular stream of walkers, bikers, and strollers circle Lafayette reservoir's shoreline. Although most of EBMUD's vast holdings are not open to the public, runners, hikers, and horseback riders have access to 68 miles trails, most of them lightly traveled, on EBMUD land.

The lands managed by EBMUD have seen significant human alteration. What were once broad valleys are now filled by dammed streams. The adjoining grasslands, once covered with native bunchgrasses, were overtaken by European annuals in the 19th century. Cattle graze the hills, keeping the grasses short and reducing shrub growth. Yet even in this modified landscape, the natural world is present: waterfowl, raptors, and other birds live near the reservoirs. Native cattails, willows, and alders thrive along shorelines, and oak, madrone, and bay laurel grow on hillsides. When running on the sweeping hills around Briones Reservoir (Run 32) or the undulating trail along Upper San Leandro Reservoir (Run 33), you will sense the remoteness of these trails and discover the "wild" East Bay.

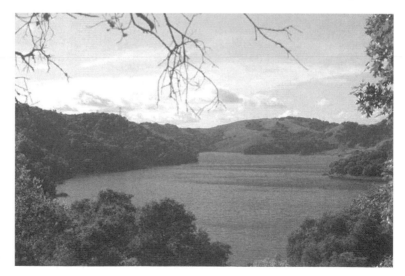

Briones Reservoir

You must have a permit to use EBMUD trails (except at Lafayette Reservoir). Permits cost $2.50 for one day, $10 for one year, or $20 for three years, and come with a trail map. You can buy a permit at the EBMUD headquarters in Orinda, at any EBMUD business office (Oakland, Richmond, San Leandro, and Walnut Creek), and at the Lafayette and San Pablo recreation areas. You can also call to request a permit application by mail. (See Appendix I for phone number.)

What You'll Find

32

BRIONES RESERVOIR

This run is a year-round treat. A rolling singletrack follows the south shore of Briones Reservoir through a cool, mixed evergreen forest. Bay laurel scents the air, water birds call near the shoreline, and the reservoir reflects billowing clouds or sparkles in the sunlight. The trail is neither too hot in the summer and fall nor too muddy in winter.

Distance	9 miles
Time	1.25–2.25 hours
Type	out-and-back
High Point/Low Point	897´/590´
Difficulty	moderate
Use	light
Maps	EBMUD trail map
Area Management	East Bay Municipal Utility District

Trailhead Access
Take the Orinda exit from Hwy. 24 and turn north on Camino Pablo. Go 2.2 miles northwest to Bear Creek Rd. Turn right and continue 4.2 miles to the Bear Creek Staging Area, on the left just past the junction with Happy Valley Rd.

Route Directions
Begin from sign-in post; follow trail across creek.
0.1 Go through metal gate and join **Bear Creek Trail.**
0.2 Turn right on gravel road.
0.3 Veer left on Bear Creek Trail.
Cross two service trails en route (closed to public access).
4.5 Overlook Staging Area; retrace steps to Bear Creek Staging Area.

About the Trail
This route begins at the eastern tip of Briones Reservoir. The narrow trail initially drops into a wooded creekbed, usually muddy in the rainy season. After a brief climb out of the creekbed you emerge on a

wide, exposed, gravel trail. Oak-studded rolling hills to the east portray a classic California scene, and rushes line the shore of the reservoir in the distance. The trail veers left before reaching the water and becomes a wide dirt path through a thriving mixed evergreen forest. Look for a spectacularly sculpted oak next to a bench.

Beneath bay laurel, oak, and madrone, the trail narrows to a singletrack and begins a gentle but steady climb up the hillside. The forest floor is rich with honeysuckle, sword fern, blackberry, soaproot, and spring-blooming hound's tongue. Across the reservoir, the water extends long amoeba-like arms into the hills.

You climb toward Bear Creek Road, enjoy a brief level stretch, and then descend again toward the reservoir. About halfway to the Overlook Staging Area, the trail follows a point of land that extends into the reservoir, and the water wraps around both sides. You can look back on your forested route and ahead to the rolling hills surrounding the reservoir.

The trail begins a gradual descent as it nears the staging area. Bunchgrasses cover open slopes where pine and oak intermingle, while coyote bush, manzanita, and chamise cast their subtle fragrance. Sticky monkeyflower blooms much of the year. A profusion of madrone trees, with smooth, rust-colored trunks, encloses the trail—subtle white blossoms decorate the trees in spring, and in fall, red berries hang in large clusters. You may notice deer tracks in the

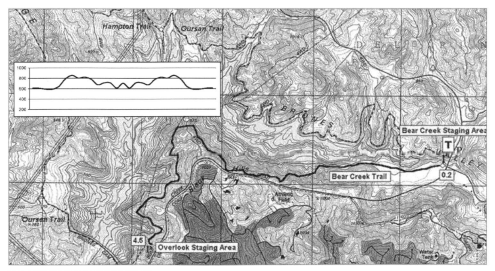

BRIONES RESERVOIR

dirt trail and hear water birds calling loudly. The trail drops close to the shore, lined by willows and rushes. To the west, San Pablo Ridge runs north-south. This barrier to summer fog keeps Contra Costa County toasty when Berkeley is ensconced in the low cloud.

At the Overlook Staging Area a narrow trail heads up a small hill to the parking lot and toilet. Retrace your steps to the Bear Valley Staging Area or check out **Alternate Routes** and continue around the reservoir.

Alternate Routes Three trails form a loop around Briones Reservoir for a challenging 14-mile run. These trails are plagued by the East Bay's sticky mud during the rainy season and summer days are often very hot, so time your run accordingly. Follow the featured route for the first 4.5 miles. At the Overlook Staging Area, continue straight ahead on the Oursan Trail and cross the dam on a paved road. Follow the arrows for the Oursan Trail, passing through a couple of metal cattle gates.

You'll enjoy sweeping views of San Pablo Reservoir and San Pablo Ridge. The trail winds in and out, following the line of several far-reaching inlets. At a junction with the Hampton Trail turn right and head back toward Briones Reservoir. You soon turn left to rejoin the Oursan Trail and follow it 5.1 miles back to the staging area.

Trail Notes
- Singletrack and service trails
- Some rocks, roots, and loose leaf cover; some mud on the Bear Valley Trail, but passable; Oursan and Hampton trails around the reservoir extremely muddy in wet weather
- No dogs
- No bikes
- Horses allowed
- Toilet at Overlook Staging Area and Bear Creek Staging Area
- No water
- No fees
- EBMUD permit required

 On Saturday mornings (May through November) between 9 AM and 1 PM the Orinda farmers market takes over a couple of blocks on Orinda Way. Satisfy yourself with fresh fruit, veggies, bread, and more.

You'll also find a Safeway and plenty of cafes and restaurants in the town of Orinda.

33

UPPER SAN LEANDRO RESERVOIR AND RIDGE LOOP

Follow EBMUD service trails along the shore of Upper San Leandro Reservoir, over exposed grassy hills and through shady oak woodland. A climb up Rocky Ridge challenges your lungs, legs, and determination. The San Leandro hills rise between this EBMUD water supply and the bay, blocking the coast's tempering climatic influence. Warm days in Berkeley and Oakland are warmer still in Moraga, and cool mornings are more likely to be frosty.

Distance	7.2 miles
Time	1-1.75 hours
Type	semi-loop
High Point/Low Point	927'/468'
Difficulty	moderate
Use	light
Maps	EBMUD trail map
Area Management	East Bay Municipal Utility District

From Hwy. 24 in Orinda, take the Orinda exit. Turn south on Moraga Way and go 4.5 miles to where it dead-ends at Moraga and Canyon roads. Turn right on Canyon Rd. After 1.2 miles, turn left into the gravel EBMUD staging area parking lot, signed VALLE VISTA.

Trailhead Access

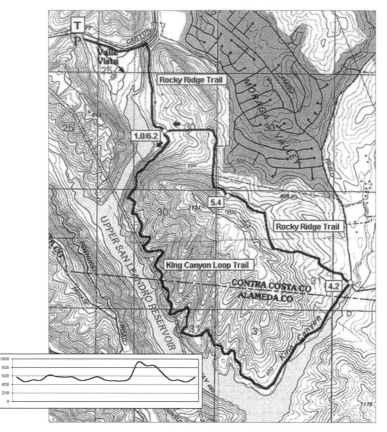

UPPER SAN LEANDRO RESERVOIR AND RIDGE LOOP

Route
Directions
Begin on **Rocky Ridge Trail.**

0.1 Veer left to stay on Rocky Ridge Trail.

0.2 Cross bridge.

1.0 Go straight on **King Canyon Loop Trail.**

2.5 Veer left at unsigned junction.

4.2 Turn left on **Rocky Ridge Trail** at EBMUD trailhead.

5.4 Turn right to continue on Rocky Ridge Trail.

5.8 Pass Old Moraga Ranch Rd. Trail.

6.2 Turn right on Rocky Ridge Trail.

About the
Trail
Upper San Leandro Reservoir is barely visible from the staging area where you begin this run. The singletrack Rocky Ridge Trail

quickly veers left and briefly parallels Canyon Road. Cross the reservoir's northern fringe on a wide wooden bridge and follow the exposed, level trail along the marshy tip of the reservoir.

You leave the Rocky Ridge Trail where it climbs steeply up the ridge (your return descent route) and continue on a gentle incline along the reservoir's eastern edge on the Kings Canyon Loop Trail. Blackberry, ferns, blue elderberry, and poison oak thrive beneath the shade of oak and bay laurel trees; coyote bush studs the open, grassy slopes. Views of the glistening waters below urge you up and down these rollercoaster hills. Across the reservoir, Redwood Park's East Ridge Trail crowns the forested hillside.

At a trail fork, veer left (the right branch dead-ends shortly). Your route then curves left (east) and borders an extension of the reservoir. Follow the trail toward King Canyon and the smooth curves of Moraga's hills. Depending on the water level, this long finger can be an emerald cove or a marshy wetland. The ridge you'll climb to return to the trailhead lies to your left, where steep grassy slopes rise to a forested ridgetop.

At another EMBUD trailhead and signpost you leave your wide trail for a singletrack and begin your ascent up the ridge. The trail at first parallels a creekbed, where oak and bay laurel offer brief segments of shade to relieve the heat of open grasslands. It then widens again into a service trail and you climb steeply and unrelentingly, passing several wide EBMUD trails (closed to the public). Just before the ridgetop you find relief when the trail turns right and heads downhill.

You see the town of Moraga in the distance, among rolling oak-studded hills that are becoming increasingly covered with houses. The trail now continues fairly level through a light forest, and then descends steeply, leveling where the Old Moraga Ranch Trail branches to the right and a house abuts the trail. You continue down the ridge on a gentler grade to complete the loop at the junction with the Kings Canyon Loop Trail. Turn right and retrace your steps to the trailhead.

Alternate Routes

If you're not up for the challenge of the Rocky Ridge Trail, the first mile of this route makes a relatively level 2-mile out-and-back run. For a little longer out-and-back, continue on the rolling trail along the reservoir for as long as you like.

Trail Notes
- Singletrack and service trails
- Mostly smooth dirt trails; sometimes rutted with dry mud; very muddy in the rainy season
- Dogs on leash on Kings Canyon Loop Trail; not allowed on Rocky Ridge Trail
- No bikes
- Horses allowed
- Toilet at trailhead; no water
- EBMUD permit required

🍴 Stop by the Sí Sí Caffé for a pick-me-up before or after your run. The small café serves coffee and espresso drinks, muffins and scones, and refreshing fruit smoothies. Go north on Country Club Drive from Canyon Road to find it. For other options, try Albertson's across the street.

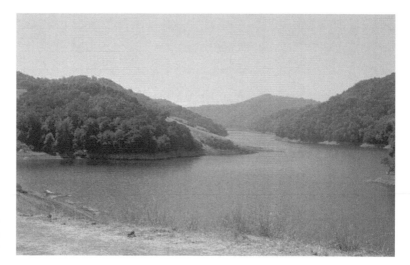

Upper San Leandro Reservoir

34

LAFAYETTE RESERVOIR

You'll find the true meaning of rollercoaster hills on Lafayette Reservoir's Rim Trail loop. Intense ups and downs over grassy, oak-studded hills make this a short but intense run; a paved loop along the shoreline is a shorter and easier option. Lafayette Reservoir is a convenient and popular spot for walkers, runners, boaters, and families. Get an early start on warm days, as this exposed trail heats up quickly.

Distance	4.7 miles
Time	0.5–1.25 hours
Type	loop
High Point/Low Point	1020′/466′
Difficulty	moderate
Use	heavy
Maps	EBMUD trail map
Area Management	East Bay Municipal Utility District

Trailhead Access

From eastbound Hwy. 24, exit at Acalanes/Mt. Diablo Blvd. From westbound Hwy. 24 exit at Acalanes/Upper Happy Valley Rd. Head east on Mt. Diablo Blvd for 0.8 mile. Turn right into Lafayette Reservoir entrance road. Follow the road to the top of the dam; park in the 2-hour meters or pay the $5 day-parking fee.

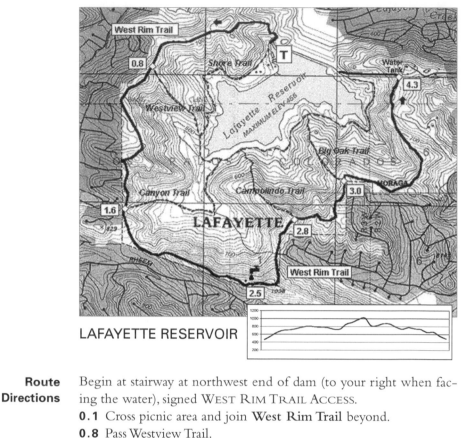

LAFAYETTE RESERVOIR

Route Directions Begin at stairway at northwest end of dam (to your right when facing the water), signed WEST RIM TRAIL ACCESS.

0.1 Cross picnic area and join **West Rim Trail** beyond.

0.8 Pass Westview Trail.

1.6 Pass Canyon Trail.
Veer right around Rheem Reservoir water tank on paved road and follow trail on left.

2.8 Pass Campolindo Trail.

3.2 Pass Big Oak Trail.

4.3 Turn left on trail signed TO VISITOR CENTER (where Sunset Trail goes straight) to return to trailhead.

About the Trail The wide, dirt West Rim Trail is smooth and well graded, but gets very muddy in the rainy season. A moderate climb to the reservoir's high rim eases you into this hilly route. Valley, black, and live oak trees cast sparse shade, and stands of coyote bush grow among grasses. The wide, sloping reservoir basin spreads below you, dotted with oaks and buckeyes. Willows, alders, sycamores, and cottonwoods line the reservoir shore. You can see your circular route ahead of you, rising and falling with the rolling hills.

Residential homes border the trail here and on much of this route. Far-reaching views also surround you on most of the run: across Hwy. 24, Briones Hills ripple northward; and Mt. Diablo rises high beyond Las Trampas and Rocky ridges in the east.

You pass the Westview and Canyon trails, which descend to the Shore Trail. Look for the raptors that often soar over these hillsides and deer tracks in the trail, and take in more views with every step. Past Rheem Reservoir (a large water tank with drinking fountain on the southeast side), you climb through pine trees to the trail's highest point. From 1038 feet you have a panoramic view—the Oakland/Berkeley hills, Briones Regional Park, Mt. Diablo, and the towns of Orinda, Moraga, and Walnut Creek.

Beyond the summit, short climbs punctuate several steep descents. You pass the Campolindo and Big Oak trails, which connect to the Shore Trail. Homes creep up the hillside to your right, and you see that you're approaching the dam and the end of this loop. Turn left and head downhill to the paved Shore Trail and to the parking lot.

Alternate Routes

The four service trails that connect the West Rim and Shore trails are good (but steep) ways to shorten or lengthen your route. If you're not up to the hills on the Rim Trail, or if you're pushing a stroller, the Shore Trail (2.8 miles) is a beautiful and satisfying loop. You also can combine the Rim and Shore trails for a 7.4-mile run.

Trail Notes

• Dirt service trail
• Wide and smooth; sticky mud in wet weather
• Dogs on leash
• No bikes on West Rim Trail; bikes (and roller/inline skates) allowed on paved shoreline trail on Tuesdays and Thursdays from noon until closing and Sundays from opening until 11 AM
• No horses
• Restrooms, water, and phone at trailhead; water at about 2.5 miles
• $5 day-parking fee, or 2-hour maximum metered parking ($0.50/hr., quarters only)
• Hours: from approximately one half hour before sunrise to one half hour after sunset
• The shoreline loop (Shore Trail) is great for strollers.

Try the house-made bread at Rising Loafer Café and Bakery on Mt. Diablo Blvd. for breakfast or lunch (outside and inside seating). Go right (east) on Mt. Diablo Blvd. for about half a mile from the reservoir road.

35

STRAWBERRY CANYON
FIRE TRAIL

Two wide canyons, Strawberry Canyon and Hamilton Gulch, run east-west from the Berkeley Hills to the campus of the University of California. You'll have views of the Campanile and beyond to San Francisco, the Golden Gate, and Mt. Tamalpais. Choose a shorter, level route or take on the full 7 miles and their accompanying hills. A white tide of fog often streams through the Golden Gate on summer mornings and afternoons, cooling this exposed trail.

Distance	7 miles
Time	1–1.75 hours
Type	out-and-back
High Point/Low Point	1333'/629'
Difficulty	moderate
Use	heavy
Maps	Trails of the East Bay Hills, Northern Section
Area Management	University of California, Berkeley

Trailhead Access

From I-80 in Berkeley exit at University Ave. Go east to the base of the UC Campus and turn left on Oxford St. Turn right at the next stoplight on Hearst St. At the second stoplight on Hearst, turn right onto Gayley Rd. Turn left at the first stop sign onto Stadium Rim Rd. Turn left at the top of the hill and the next stop sign onto Centennial Dr. Pass the UC Botanical Garden and the Lawrence Hall of Science. Turn right into the Space Sciences Institute and continue to the second parking lot on the left. The trail begins at the far end of the lot, marked by a blue fire trail sign. NOTE: You must have a UC Berkeley permit to park in this lot from 9 AM to 5 PM, Monday through Friday.

Alternate parking: Continue on Centennial Dr. past the Space Sciences Institute. At the stop sign, cross Grizzly Peak Rd. onto Golf Course Dr. Turn right into the gravel parking area. Park here and walk south 0.2 mile on Grizzly Peak to the metal fire-trail gate and the beginning of this run. You can also park along the street on Grizzly Peak Blvd. closer to the metal gate.

Yet another option is to begin this run at the other end. Park in a lot on Centennial Dr., 0.4 mile from your turn onto Centennial Dr.

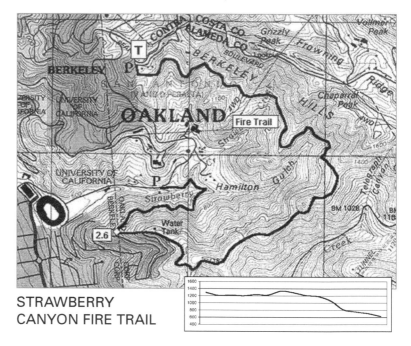

STRAWBERRY CANYON FIRE TRAIL

Route Directions Begin on wide fire trail at edge of parking lot (or at metal gate on Grizzly Peak, depending on where you parked).

0.2 Mileage post

0.7 Mileage post

1.7 Bench

2.5 Steep connecter trail between upper and lower fire trails.

2.6 Turn right at bottom of hill to continue on fire trail.

3.5 Centennial Dr. Retrace route to trailhead.

About the Trail A wide fire trail hugs the rim of Strawberry Canyon and Hamilton Gulch, and then descends into the shady ravine: the upper trail offers 1.5 level miles plus a 1.0-mile descent; a steep path connects to a lower trail that gradually descends for another mile. You decide how far and how hard you want to go.

The trail begins among eucalyptus trees that provide shade for the first half mile or so, their fragrance especially strong when the ridge is smothered in moist fog. In wet months, Strawberry Creek descends the hillside above you through a tangle of vegetation and crosses underneath the trail into the canyon. Views of the bay peek through thinning eucalyptus, and in spring the deep blue blossoms of blue dicks grace this hillside, later accompanied by lupine and Indian paintbrush.

After just under a mile, the trail curves sharply to the left and traces the curve of another canyon, Hamilton Gulch. Across the wide breach you can see the continuation of your route. Before you, chaparral-covered slopes rise toward Grizzly Peak. Interesting rock formations jut from these slopes, surrounded by deep green vegetation in winter and spring and by golden grasses in summer and fall. In spring, blue lupine, bright orange Indian paintbrush, and yellow sticky monkeyflower add bright spots of color to the hillsides.

Two more creeks pass underneath the trail as it continues on a level route along the upper edge of the canyon. Full and rushing after heavy winter rains, they are barely noticeable the rest of the year. Your views stretch through the canyon to the University of California, Berkeley campus (you may be able to read the time on the campanile clock) and beyond to a glistening San Francisco; Mt. Tamalpais looms high in Marin, and Alcatraz and Angel islands rise in the bay.

After several gentle bends and short straight-aways, you reach a bench, which marks a good turnaround point for a level run. As the trail descends into the canyon, the temperature drops a couple of degrees. In fall, white snowberries hang from bushes along the trail; the pink blossoms of currants cover the hillsides in winter and release a strong, spicy fragrance. Hazelnut and sticky monkeyflower grow abundantly.

A steep path links the upper and lower fire trails; the narrow trail on the right is less steep. The lower fire trail descends gradually, in the partial shade of bay laurel and oak, and ferns, hazelnut, blackberry, and currants line the banks. The trail crosses culverts over Strawberry Creek at the southern boundary of the University of California Botanical Gardens and ends just beyond at Centennial Drive. Retrace your steps to the trailhead at the upper end of Centennial Drive.

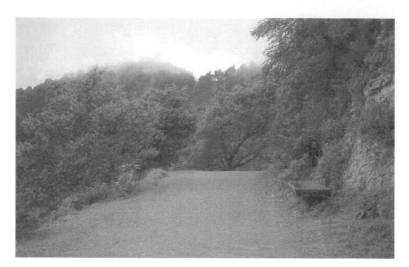

Strawberry
Canyon
Fire Trail

**Alternate
Routes**
Since this is an out-and-back trail, make your run as long or short as you like. If you don't want to run the steep connector between the upper and lower fire trails, you can do a 5-mile roundtrip run and still get in one good hill.

This also is a great route to combine with trails in Tilden Regional Park (Runs 22 and 23). Cross Grizzly Peak Blvd. to Golf Course Drive and explore the trails that begin from the parking lot and trailhead there.

Trail Notes
• Fire trail
• Smooth dirt trail; sticky mud in wet weather
• Dogs off-leash
• No bikes
• Horses allowed
• No toilet or water
• No fees
• Popular with runners and walkers, especially dog owners

 The area around the UC campus has numerous restaurants and coffee shops. On the northside, choose from an array of inexpensive eateries on Euclid Avenue at Hearst. On the southside of campus, you can take your pick from the many options along Bancroft Avenue.

Non-native plants have almost taken over this University of California Ecological Study Area. Eucalyptus trees abound, as well as French broom, the most widespread pest plant in California. French broom seriously threatens native plant species, because it spreads rapidly and crowds out other vegetation. Nevertheless, the bright yellow flowers that appear each spring are colorful and sweet-smelling.

You'll hear rather than see another exotic on this trail: the strange sounds that echo across the canyon are laughing hyenas. Since the mid-1980s, these spotted hyenas from Kenya have lived in captivity in the Berkeley Hills as part of a university study on aggression and sexual dominance.

36

JOAQUIN MILLER LOOP

This is a fast route with one climb and one downhill. Most of the run winds along a flat, smooth trail through a shady redwood forest. On a clear day sunlight filters through the redwoods, and expansive views of the bay and the Golden Gate meet you at every opening. When fog shrouds these hills, the redwood forest becomes a misty haven, removed from the homes that border it.

Distance	3.6 miles
Time	0.5-1 hour
Type	loop
High Point/Low Point	1432′/952′
Difficulty	easy
Use	heavy
Maps	Trails of the East Bay Hills, Northern Section
Area Management	City of Oakland, Department of Parks, Recreation, and Cultural Affairs

Trailhead Access From Hwy. 13 northbound in Oakland, take the Joaquin Miller Rd./Lincoln Ave. exit. Turn right onto Joaquin Miller Rd., and continue 0.8 mile to Sanborn Dr., the park entrance. (Don't be confused by the gated Sanborn Dr. you pass before reaching the one you're looking for.) Turn left and go 0.1 mile to the ranger station parking area on the left.

From Hwy. 13 southbound, take the Joaquin Miller Rd./Lincoln Ave. exit. Stay left and at a stop sign turn left onto Monterey Blvd. Turn left again at the stoplight immediately afterward onto Joaquin Miller Rd., then follow the directions above.

To find the trailhead, walk back on Sanborn Dr. toward Joaquin Miller Dr. The trail begins beyond the yellow gate at the signboard with map.

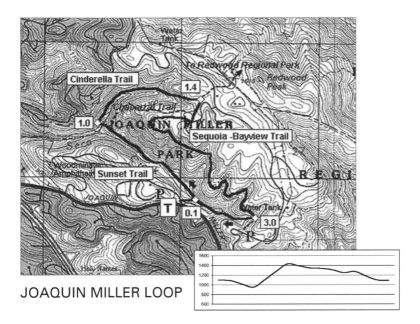

JOAQUIN MILLER LOOP

Route Directions

Begin at yellow metal gate and signboard. Go straight on wide trail, past small dirt path on left to picnic area.

0.1 Turn left on **Sunset Trail**.

0.2 Pass Sunset Loop Trail.

1.0 Turn right on **Cinderella Trail**.

1.4 Turn right on **Sequoia-Bay View Trail**. (You've gone too far if you meet the paved path, just a few yards beyond.)

Stay right on Sequoia–Bay View Trail.

Pass Chaparral Trail.

3.0 Turn right on **Sunset Trail**.

About the Trail

You begin on the Sunset Trail, a wide, smooth path that descends gently through redwood trees. As you approach the creekbed, you pass a bathroom building, a picnic area, and then a stone bridge. Palo Seco Creek parallels the trail and, unlike its name, is not a dry stick but a well-endowed stream, flanked by willows, redwoods, coast live oak, and big-leaf maple.

You leave the shade of the redwoods and continue on the level trail, flanked by blackberries and abundant French broom, which produces sweet smells and bright yellow flowers in late winter and spring. The trail narrows to a singletrack and passes the Chaparral Trail.

Where the trail dips into the ravine of the creek, you turn onto the easy-to-miss Cinderella Trail (the sign is obscured by brush) and begin the only climb of the route, next to a tributary of Palo Seco Creek. French broom predominates but bay laurel, willows, coyote bush, and cow parsnip make this a beautiful little singletrack. The Sequoia-Bay View Trail turnoff is an unsigned, narrow path that heads sharply right as you crest the ridge, and is the only trail that branches off the Cinderella Trail.

Follow the narrow, brushy path (Sequoia-Bay View signs will soon reassure you that you're on the right track) and pass the other end of the Chaparral Trail. Your trail broadens and levels as it winds through a redwood forest, dipping into lush ravines and opening to vistas of San Francisco and the Golden Gate. Huckleberry, snowberry, poison oak, and ferns thrive beneath the redwoods. You pass four adjoining trails: Horse Arena, Fern Ravine, Wild Rose, and Big Trees. As you near the Sunset Trail, oak and bay laurel prevail and a spectacular view of the East Bay and San Francisco spreads through a break in the trees.

You turn right on the Sunset Trail and descend the root-studded path, beneath dense redwoods. The trail shortly levels and passes a picnic area before it returns to the trailhead.

Alternate Routes Joaquin Miller Park's proximity to Redwood Park makes for some excellent extended routes. At the top of the Cinderella Trail, instead of turning right on the Sequoia-Bay View Trail, continue to the parking lot just beyond the turnoff. Run through the parking lot and carefully cross Skyline Blvd. Follow the paved road to the Chabot Space and Science Center to the West Ridge Trail. Turn left or right to hook up with the network of trails in Redwood Park. See the Redwood Park routes (Runs 24 and 25) for ideas.

Trail Notes • Fire and singletrack trails
• Cinderella Trail is narrow; some roots and rocks on second part of Sunset Trail; some muddy sections
• Dogs on leash; no dogs in picnic areas
• Bikes and horses allowed on all trails on this route
• Toilets and water at trailhead
• No fees
• Ranger station has maps and information about the park's geology and trees. Open every day from 9 AM to 5 PM.

PENINSULA TRAIL RUNS

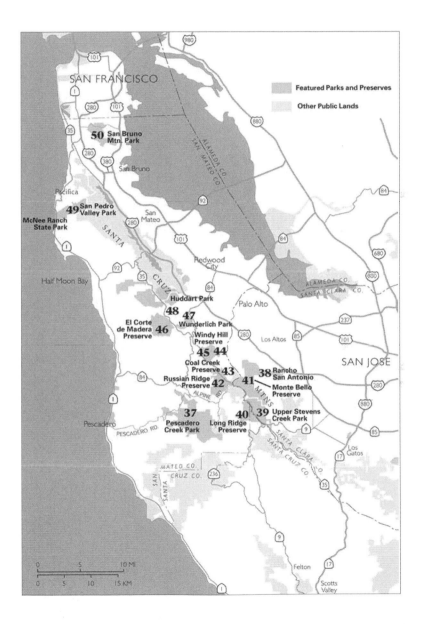

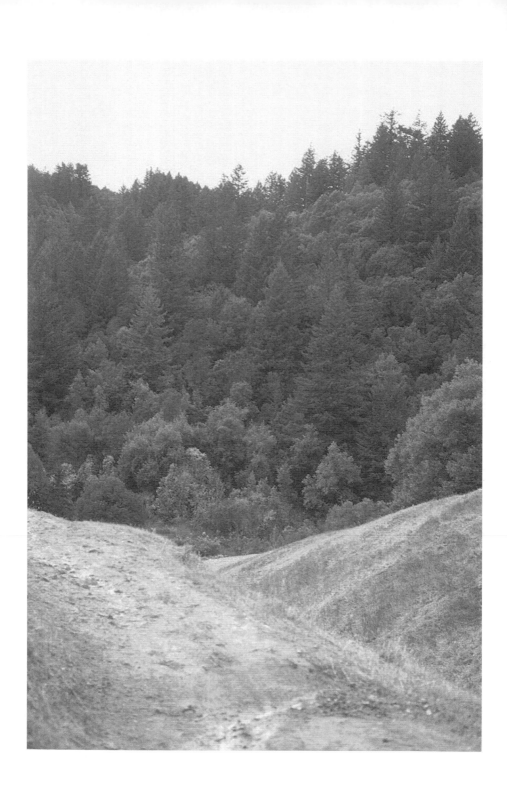

PENINSULA

LAY OF THE LAND

The long, protective arm of the San Francisco Peninsula reaches south from the city of San Francisco and wraps around the lowland of the South Bay. It is marked in its entirety by the Santa Cruz Mountains (part of the Coast Range), that rise between the ocean and the bay, from San Bruno Mountain in the north to the Gabilan Range near Monterey Bay. Acting as a barrier to the maritime climate, the mountains create distinctly different landscapes on the coastal and interior slopes. On the eastern (inland) flank, creeks cut deep canyons and high ridges as they flow toward the bay; oak, bay laurel, alder, and big-leaf maple trees border the watercourses on these steep slopes. On the west side, grassy slopes cascade more gently toward the coast; redwoods (all second- or third-growth) thrive on the often-foggy hillsides, and Douglas-fir, oak, and bay laurel intermingle in the forests. Several creeks, larger than those on the eastern slope due to heavier rainfall, empty into the Pacific.

The San Andreas fault is a defining feature of the peninsula, entering land at Mussel Rock in Daly City and continuing south, parallel to the Santa Cruz Mountains. The mountains rise to the west of the fault, and lower Monte Bello Ridge, topped by 2810-foot Black Mountain, lies to the east. Stevens Creek flows through fault's deep canyon. The San Andreas fault divides the Pacific and North American plates, and as the Pacific plate inches northwest, land west of the fault moves with it.

Thousands of acres on the peninsula are protected as parks and open space, ensuring that the land will remain undeveloped and accessible for recreationists and nature-lovers. Trailheads line Skyline Blvd. (Hwy. 35), along the ridge of the Santa Cruz Mountains, and provide access to county parks and open space preserves east and west of the crest. Highway 1 runs along the peninsula's coast, offering stunning views for travelers and providing access to sandy beaches for beachcombers and surfers.

Opposite page:
Long Ridge OSP
(Runs 39 and 40)

229

PESCADERO CREEK COUNTY PARK

Forty miles of trails traverse forested slopes and follow cool creekbeds in Pescadero Creek County Park, one component of a cluster of parks in the drainage basin of Pescadero Creek. Its 6486 acres lie between Sam McDonald and Memorial County parks and abut Portola Redwoods State Park. The network of trails though these parks offer short, simple runs as well as challenging loops.

Densely forested Butano Ridge (2,000 feet) rises from the southern banks of the deep bed of Pescadero Creek. On the opposite side, sparse woodlands and grassy hillsides cover Towne Ridge (1,200 feet).

What You'll Find

Pescadero Creek County Park is open from 8 AM to sunset. Dogs are not allowed in the park. Bikes are allowed only on Old Haul Road. Horses are allowed on all park trails.

Toilets and water are both available at the Memorial County Park campground and ranger station. Park maps are available at the ranger station—0.25 mile west of Wurr Road. There is a $4/parking fee at Memorial County Park ranger station.

37

OLD HAUL ROAD

The cool canyon of Pescadero Creek is a welcome escape from summer heat and is just far enough from the coast (about 7 miles) to often be free of fog. Follow this old logging road for up to 5.7 miles—to where it meets Portola Redwoods State Park.

Distance	up to 11.4 miles
Time	up to 3 hours
Type	out-and-back
High Point/Low Point	588′/293′
Difficulty	easy to strenuous
Use	light
Maps	map at ranger station
Area Management	San Mateo County Parks

Trailhead Access

From Hwy. 84 (La Honda Rd.) in La Honda, on the west side of Skyline Blvd., turn left (southeast) on Pescadero Rd. Go 1.1 miles to the intersection with Alpine Rd. Make a sharp right to stay on Pescadero Rd. and continue 4.5 miles to Wurr Rd. Turn left. The Hoffman Creek Trailhead is 0.5 mile ahead on the left.

From Hwy. 1, turn left on Pescadero Rd. After 11 miles, turn right on Wurr Rd. The Hoffman Creek Trailhead is 0.5 mile ahead on the left.

The ranger station, where you can pick up a map, is 0.25 mile west of Wurr Rd., signed for Memorial County Park.

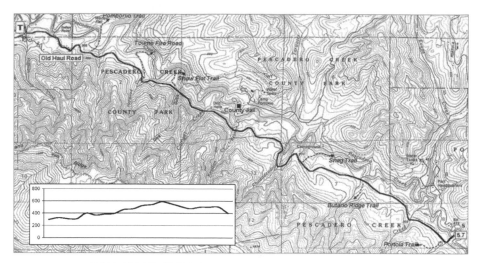

OLD HAUL ROAD

Route Directions

NOTE: Other than the total, distances are estimates.

Begin on **Old Haul Rd.**

Pass Pomponio Trail.

Pass Towne Fire Rd.

2.0 Pass Shaw Flat Trail.

   Pass Butano Ridge Loop Trail.

   Pass Snag Trail.

4.5 Pass Butano Ridge Loop Trail.

5.7 Portola Trail, Portola State Park.

About the Trail

From the parking area turn left (east) and cross the wooden bridge. A signpost and map stand in the clearing on the other side. Fruit trees ring the edges of the meadow—the remains of an old orchard—and thick redwoods rise to the high ridges.

The wide, dirt Old Haul Road trail sets off through the clearing and soon dips into redwoods. The shady forest will keep you cool the entire route. Dense groves of alder punctuate the redwoods and ferns grow on the moist hillsides. The trail rolls up and down on easy grades, and the asphalt surface from the road's logging days occasionally appears.

The Towne Fire Road and the Shaw Flat Trail branch left and cross Pescadero Creek to reach Shaw Flat Trail Camp. Just beyond, the Butano Ridge Loop Trail heads up the ridge to the right. You stay on Old Haul Road and pass numerous creeks that drain from the hillside into the deep ravine far below you to the left. Look for Keystone Creek's small waterfall that cascades down the moist hillside.

The San Mateo County Jail is situated in the middle of Pescadero Creek County Park; don't be alarmed if you hear the jail loudspeaker once you get about halfway along Old Haul Road.

Shortly beyond signed Rhododendron Creek, the Snag Trail branches right, a shortcut to the Bridge Trail. Old Haul Road descends after Hooker Creek to the other end of the Butano Ridge Loop Trail. Just before the end of Old Haul Road, you meet the Portola Trail and Portola State Park Road—a good turnaround point if you haven't turned around already.

Alternate Routes

You can explore some great loops in Pescadero Creek County Park, with two caveats: the disconcerting but harmless county jail, and wet feet. An approximately 10-mile loop leaves Old Haul Road at the Snag Trail and crosses the creek to return to the trailhead on the Pomponio Trail. The route crosses a paved road that leads to the county jail. On this loop—and on a shorter one that turns right on the Shaw Flat Trail—you may have to resort to taking your shoes off to cross the creek, unless the water is very low. There is no bridge.

Trail Notes

- Wide former logging road
- No dogs
- Bikes allowed on Old Haul Road
- Horses allowed
- No water at trailhead or trail camps along the route; toilet and water at Memorial County Park ranger station; toilets at Shaw Flat and Tarwater trail camps (slightly off featured route)
- No fees at Wurr Road trailhead

The coastal town of Pescadero, a few miles west on Pescadero Creek Road, is a fun place to get picnic supplies. Don't miss the Garlic Herb Artichoke Bread from Arcangeli Grocery Company/Norm's Market on Main Street. The bread itself makes this run worth the trip.

MIDPENINSULA REGIONAL OPEN SPACE DISTRICT

Midpeninsula Regional Open Space District preserves dot the San Francisco Peninsula, from valley lowlands to the crest of the Santa Cruz Mountains, and range in size from 55 to more than 14,000 acres. The 24 open space areas that the district manages serve many functions for the Bay Area community, providing scenic beauty, protecting native plant and animal habitats, and helping to contain urban sprawl.

MROSD was created in 1972 when voters approved an initiative placed on the ballot by peninsula conservationists. From modest initial holdings in Santa Clara County, the MROSD greenbelt expanded significantly over three decades to include land in 16 cities in San Mateo, Santa Clara, and Santa Cruz counties. MROSD trails link many preserves, and even more are linked by long-distance trails like the Bay Area Ridge Trail and the Skyline-to-the-Sea Trail.

What You'll Find

MROSD works to keep the preserves as natural as possible to protect the land and animal habitats; to this end, the district provides only the most basic amenities. Most preserves have a toilet at the trailhead, but no water. All preserves are open daily, from dawn until one-half hour after sunset. Dogs are allowed on certain trails, but must be on a maximum 6-foot leash at all times. Horses are allowed on many trails in the preserves. Check with individual preserves for guidelines.

MROSD identifies trailheads along Skyline Blvd. with an abbreviation of the preserve name and a number. For example, El Corte de Madera Open Space Preserve has four trailheads: the northernmost one, across the road from Skeggs Point, is called CM01, where the Tafoni Trail begins; CM02 is 0.7 mile south, the Methuselah trailhead; CM03 and CM04 follow in succession to the south.

38

RANCHO SAN ANTONIO

The steep slopes of Black Mountain tower above Rancho San Antonio and dive into the deep ravine of Wildcat Canyon, the heart of the preserve. On this loop, you'll feel far from the crowds and subdivisions around the trailhead. You circle the canyon on wide trails along moist creekbeds, across wildflower-dotted hillsides, and up and down oak- and bay laurel-shaded slopes.

Distance	9.8 miles
Time	1.25 – 2.5 hours
Type	loop
High Point/Low Point	1536′/363′
Difficulty	moderate
Use	heavy
Maps	MROSD map at trailhead
Area Management	Midpeninsula Regional Open Space District

Trailhead Access

From Hwy. 280 in Mountain View take the Foothill Expressway exit. Turn right on Cristo Rey Dr. After 1 mile turn left into the county park entrance. Stay left, following signs to restrooms, and park in the far northwest parking lot.

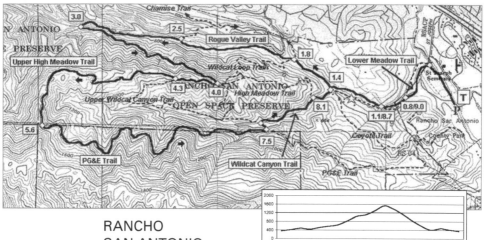

RANCHO
SAN ANTONIO

Route Directions

Begin at northwest corner of northwest parking lot.
Cross bridge and turn right on trail signed to DEER HOLLOW FARM.

0.5 Go straight on **Lower Meadow Trail** from MROSD preserve sign.

0.8 Cross paved road and follow signs to Rogue Valley Trail.

1.1 Meet paved road again and turn right; go through farm.

1.4 Join **Rogue Valley Trail**; pass turnoff to High Meadow Trail.

1.8 Pass Wildcat Loop Trail.

2.5 Pass turnoff to Chamise Trail.

3.0 Turn left; continue on Rogue Valley Trail.

4.0 Turn right, signed to Upper Wildcat Canyon Trail.

4.3 Go straight on **Upper High Meadow Trail,** past Upper Wildcat Canyon Trail.

5.6 Veer left on **PG&E Trail,** signed 4 MILES TO COUNTY PARK.

7.5 Turn left, 0.1 TO WILDCAT CANYON TRAIL.

7.6 Turn right on **Wildcat Canyon Trail** to Deer Hollow Farm.

8.1 Pass High Meadow Trail.
Veer right on **Farm Bypass Trail.** Stay right at next junction.

8.4 Veer left toward preserve entrance. (Coyote Trail goes right.)

8.7 Cross wooden bridge and paved road. Retrace steps to parking area.

About the Trail

The county park parking lot, the only available non-permit parking, is about a half mile from the MROSD preserve entrance. Cross the bridge at the far northwestern edge of the parking lot and turn right on a wide, gravelly path, following signs to Deer Hollow Farm. You skirt a large grass field and tennis courts and then cross a paved road to an MROSD preserve sign, where you can pick up a trail map.

Begin on the Lower Meadow Trail, here wide dirt path, and follow it through the farm, where you'll pass goats, sheep, and chickens in pens alongside turn-of-the-century ranch buildings. Look for signs directing you to the Rogue Valley Trail. Beyond the farm, the level dirt trail follows slender Rogue Valley beside a willow-lined creek. A steep hillside, thick with live oak and bay laurel, keeps the trail cool and shaded. Red toyon berries abound in fall and winter. Vibrant green moss grows on tree trunks and across the creek, coyote bush, chamise, and oaks grow on drier slopes.

You climb gently, and soon pass a small pond, dry in some seasons, where the stream was dammed. Beyond, blackberry grows thick along the trail, and tall big-leaf maple drop golden leaves on the trail in fall.

The Rogue Valley Trail turns left sharply and doubles back on a steady but gentle climb up the hillside above the valley. Honeysuckle vines dangle from madrone branches and bay laurel trees fill shady gullies. As you climb higher, you have views of the South Bay and the Diablo Range beyond.

On a low ridgetop, you reach the Upper High Meadow Trail, where open slopes boast spring wildflowers—blue dicks, lupine, blue-eyed grass, and mule ears. Below, Wildcat Canyon cuts a deep ravine between you and the steep eastern flank of Black Mountain. The PG&E Trail, your return route, cuts a sloping line on the rippled hillside across the canyon. You climb gently up the exposed Upper High Meadow Trail, past grassy slopes dotted with coyote bush and chamise.

You wrap around the eastern side of a knoll and take in north-stretching views of the South Bay. The trail levels beneath a thick canopy of oak trees and begins to curve as it rounds the canyon head. Bay laurel and toyon line a last steep climb to meet the PG&E Trail, where a sign points left 4.0 miles to the county park. (On this route, you will leave the PG&E Trail in 2.1 miles to return through the preserve.)

On the gravelly dirt trail you begin to lose the elevation you just gained; level sections and gentle rises are welcome breaks for your knees from the occasional steep sections. On either side of the wide, shelf-like trail the hillside is covered in chamise, coyote bush, toyon, oak, and bay laurel. On clear winter days, views down the canyon of the South Bay and the Diablo Range beyond are especially spectacular. Not so spectacular are the pink subdivisions just beyond the park boundary. Look to the High Meadow Trail on the grassy slopes above the other side of the canyon.

You turn left on a singletrack trail, signed to WILDCAT CANYON TRAIL, and descend switchbacks into the canyon. On the floor, the trail descends slightly along a seasonal creek and crosses back and forth over the creek on several wooden bridges. The moist ravine is shaded by oak, buckeye, big-leaf maple, and skinny, green-trunked bay laurel, reaching high for the light.

Instead of backtracking through the farm, veer off on the Farm Bypass Trail signed to the county park; it will shortly deliver you to the Lower Meadow Trail, about a mile before the MROSD preserve trailhead.

Alternate Routes The 23 miles of trails at this convenient and popular preserve offer a variety of routes—challenging and easy, shady and exposed—along creeks and across open slopes. For a shorter route, and to avoid the steepest parts of the preserve, tackle a loop on the Wildcat Loop Trail and High Meadow Trail or Wildcat Canyon Trail.

Trail Notes • Mostly fire trails; one singletrack
• Wide, smooth dirt trails; gravelly trails are good after rains
• No dogs
• No bikes allowed beyond Deer Hollow Farm
• Horses allowed on Rogue Valley, High Meadow, Upper High Meadow, and PG&E trails
• Restrooms, water, and phone at trailhead; toilets at Deer Hollow Farm
• No fees
• Popular preserve, although the trails are much less crowded than the parking lot

39

GRIZZLY FLAT LOOP

The best of the eastern and western flanks of the Santa Cruz Mountains: coastal and Diablo Range views, oak and bay-laurel forests, and creek crossings, all accessed by intimate singletracks and smooth fire roads.

Distance	10.2 miles
Time	1.5–2.5 hours
Type	loop
High Point/Low Point	2612′/1295′
Difficulty	strenuous
Use	light
Maps	MROSD map at trailhead
Area Management	Midpeninsula Regional Open Space District and Upper Stevens Creek County Park

Trailhead Access

Take Page Mill Rd. from Palo Alto, Woodside/La Honda Rd. (Hwy. 84) from Woodside, or Hwy. 92 to Skyline Blvd. Go south on Skyline and pass the Grizzly Flat trailhead, about 3 miles south of Page Mill Rd. Continue about 1.7 miles to Long Ridge Open Space Preserve gate LR 01 and park on the side of the road. The trailhead is on the west side of Skyline Blvd.

Route Directions

Begin at LR 01 on signed Bay Area Ridge Trail Route. Turn right on **Hickory Oaks Trail.**

0.2 Veer left on singletrack detour (signed BAY AREA RIDGE TRAIL).

0.3 Rejoin Hickory Oaks Trail.

0.8 Stay right on singletrack to Ward Rd.; Hickory Oak Trail goes left.

1.0 Join **Ward Rd.** and continue straight.

1.1 Turn right on **Peters Creek Trail** at junction with Ward and Long Ridge roads.

1.6 Turn left to continue on Peters Creek Trail. Stay right at junctions on Peters Creek Trail, following signs to Grizzly Flat parking area.

3.2 Cross Skyline Blvd. to **Grizzly Flat parking area** and Stevens Creek Park. Take left-hand trail, signed 2 MILES TO GRIZZLY FLAT TRAIL.

4.0 Pass right-branching trail that leads to Grizzly Flat Trail.

5.0 Grizzly Flat Trail joins from right.

5.2 From Grizzly Flat Trail turn left on singletrack, signed 0.5 MILE TO CANYON TRAIL.

5.4 Cross creek.

5.7 Turn right on **Canyon Trail.**

6.0 Veer right on **Table Mountain Trail.** Canyon Trail to Stevens Canyon Rd. goes left.

6.1 Cross creek.

7.1 Turn right on unsigned **Charcoal Rd.**

7.2 Veer right on singletrack signed for foot traffic only.

9.9 Rejoin Charcoal Rd. and turn right on **Bay Area Ridge Trail.**

About the Trail

Go up a short hill from the trailhead to join the unsigned Hickory Oaks Trail. Turn right and climb on the wide, rock-strewn trail, beneath tall oak trees. Shortly after the crest of the hill, veer left on a small singletrack that rounds a grassy knob. You take in your first expansive view of the coastline on this short detour. The narrow trail wraps back to rejoin the Hickory Oaks Trail, and you follow the broad, smooth trail as it rolls along the ridgeline and wraps around grassy knolls.

Say goodbye to coastal views and veer right on a singletrack trail where Hickory Oaks turns left: yours is a shorter route to Ward Road. Your singletrack meets unpaved Ward Road and descends to a

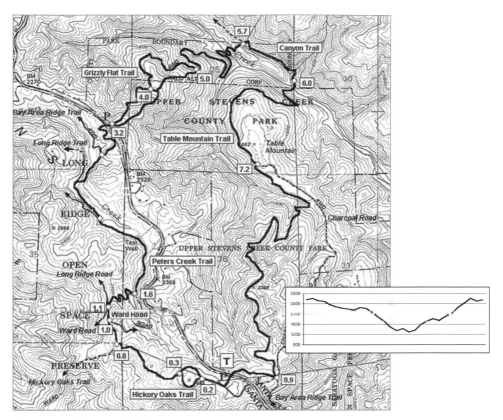

GRIZZLY FLAT LOOP

junction, where a green street sign marks Ward and Long Ridge roads. You turn left on the singletrack Peters Creek Trail and leave the ridge via switchbacks. Private property abuts the reserve at the base of the ridge. You cross Peters Creek on a dam that has created a small upstream pond.

The smooth dirt trail follows the creek for the next mile or so; stay right at junctions, heading for the Grizzly Flat parking area. You pass beneath oak and bay laurel and through grassy fields dotted with coyote bush. Moss covers jumbled boulders in the creekbed and ferns thrive in the moisture. After crossing a wooden bridge you begin a gentle climb out of the low canyon to Skyline Blvd. and the Grizzly Flat parking area.

Across Skyline Blvd. you enter Stevens Creek Park. Two trails leave from the trailhead and parallel each other to meet at Grizzly

Flat; take the left-hand trail, signed 2 MILES TO THE GRIZZLY FLAT TRAIL. Descend the gentle grade beneath Douglas-fir, oak, bay laurel, and madrone; sunlight scatters patterns on occasional twigs and rocks on the wide trail. You pass two trails on your right—connectors to the Grizzly Flat Trail. The sound of the creek signals your approach to the canyon bottom, and cool air rises to greet you as the trail switchbacks into the ravine.

At Grizzly Flat you turn left to follow a level singletrack to the creek. Make your way across—there is no bridge, so in high water you may get your feet a little wet. The narrow trail climbs gradual switchbacks up the opposite bank in the deep shade of bay laurel. You meet the Canyon Trail, a popular route through Stevens Creek Canyon from Monte Bello Preserve to Stevens Canyon Road, and turn right to descend through this cool, shaded canyon on a rocky trail.

Soon you turn off on the singletrack Table Mountain Trail. After another bridgeless creek crossing, you climb back out of the canyon. Switchbacks lead up a fern-covered hillside to a wooden bridge that spans a deep gully. The smooth dirt trail then rolls gently up and down along the side of the canyon, high above the distant sound of the creek. Look for brilliant orange-yellow mushrooms growing in the moist ground. As you approach Table Mountain, the change in vegetation reflects the drier conditions. You pass holly-leaf cherry bushes, coyote bush, honeysuckle, and madrone, and emerge on a grassy knoll; the high, forested ridge rises to your right.

Your trail meets wide Charcoal Road, and after a short flat stretch, you veer right on an alternate singletrack trail for foot traffic only. On a gentle-to-moderate nearly three-mile climb, you reach Skyline Blvd. Madrone, Douglas-fir, and oak shade stretches of the route; from exposed plateaus, you catch glimpses of Monte Bello Ridge (behind you across Stevens Creek Canyon) and the Diablo Range through tall stands of manzanita, shrub oak, and chamise. To return to the trailhead go north on the Bay Area Ridge Trail from the second junction with Charcoal Road. (The Ridge Trail continues south to Saratoga Gap. See below.)

Alternate Routes To extend this route, begin your run at Saratoga Gap (at the junction of Hwys. 35 and 9) and run 1.7 miles on the Skyline Trail (also the Bay Area Ridge Trail) to join this route at Charcoal Road. For shorter routes in this area, see the Long Ridge Open Space Preserve (Run 40).

- Singletrack and fire trails **Trail Notes**
- Some roots and rocks on Hickory Oaks Trail; two creek crossings— may be difficult in high water
- Dogs allowed for 0.4 mile in Long Ridge Preserve
- Bikes allowed on Grizzly Flat, Canyon, and Table Mountain trails (uphill only on Table Mountain); no bikes on singletrack along Charcoal Road
- Horses allowed on all trails except singletrack along Charcoal Road
- No toilet or water
- No fees
- Hours: Long Ridge Open Space Preserve, dawn to one-half hour after sunset; Upper Stevens Creek County Park, 8 AM to dusk

40

LONG RIDGE LOOP

Begin and end this semi-loop in a cool creekside canyon crowded with lush ferns, vibrant green moss, and riparian willows; then follow the Bay Area Ridge Trail on singletrack and fire roads through open grasslands that overlook the panorama of the Santa Cruz Mountains and the Pescadero Creek watershed.

Distance	7.4 miles
Time	1–2 hours
Type	semi-loop
High Point/Low Point	2568′/2153′
Difficulty	moderate
Use	light
Maps	MROSD map at trailhead
Area Management	Midpeninsula Regional Open Space District

Trailhead Access Take Page Mill Rd. from Palo Alto, Woodside/La Honda Rd. (Hwy. 84) from Woodside, or Hwy. 92 to Skyline Blvd. Go south on Skyline Blvd. to the Grizzly Flat roadside parking area, on the east side of the road, about 3 miles south of Page Mill Rd. Long Ridge Preserve trailhead is on west side of Skyline Blvd.

Route Directions

0.4 Veer left on **Peters Creek Trail** and the Bay Area Ridge Trail south; Bay Area Ridge Trail also goes north to Skyline Open Space Preserve.

0.5 Pass right-branching Long Ridge Trail.

0.9 Pass right-branching trail to Long Ridge.

1.2 Pass side trails to Skyline Blvd.

1.6 Turn right at preserve boundary.

2.1 Turn left sharply on (upper) **Ward Rd.**

2.2 Veer right to **Hickory Oaks Trail.**

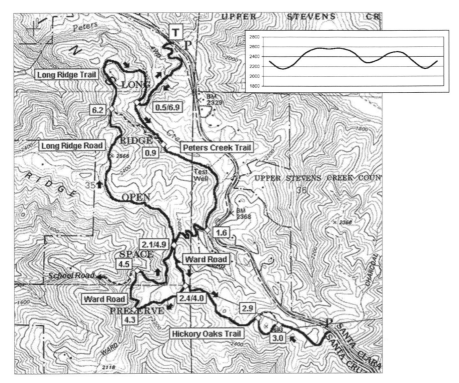

LONG RIDGE LOOP

2.4 Continue straight (left) on **Hickory Oaks Trail.**
2.9 Turn right on singletrack detour.
3.0 Rejoin Hickory Oaks Trail.
3.2 Turn around at Skyline Blvd.
4.0 Veer left on Hickory Oaks Trail (also Ward Rd).
4.3 Turn right on **Ward Rd.** at junction with Ranch Spring Trail.
4.5 Continue straight on Ward Rd. at junction with School Rd.
4.9 Go straight on **Long Ridge Rd.** at fork in Ward Rd.
5.4 Veer right on **Long Ridge Trail.**
6.2 Pass trail to Peters Creek Trail.
6.9 Turn left on **Peters Creek Trail** (also Bay Area Ridge Trail).
7.0 Veer right, to Grizzly Flat parking.

About the Trail

A narrow singletrack descends from the trailhead on Skyline ridge into Peters Creek Canyon, across grassy open hills and through a Douglas-fir, bay laurel, oak, and madrone forest. Just past a junction with the northern extension of the Bay Area Ridge Trail, you cross a wooden bridge over the small streambed of Peters Creek, lined by snowberry and willows. Head south on the Peters Creek Trail (also Bay Area Ridge Trail) along the broadening bed of the creek, where bay-laurel branches arch over ferns and moss-covered boulders. You leave the creek after a gentle climb and enter an open meadow surrounded by trees. Your smooth dirt trail follows the general route of the creek for the next mile, beneath bay laurel and oaks, and through coyote bush-dotted grasslands. You pass a short spur to the Long Ridge Trail and a couple of small trails that branch left to Skyline Blvd.

At the preserve boundary, you turn right and cross a dammed section of the creek on a wooden bridge. Beyond, gentle switchbacks climb to Long Ridge, beneath oak and madrone. In fall, look for bright red rosehips on wild rose bushes that grow along the trail. Go through a wooden gate at the ridgeline, where your first coastal views greet you. A street sign on a metal pole indicates Long Ridge Road to the right and Ward Road to the left. Go left on the upper fork of wide Ward Road and follow it to a right-branching single-track trail that cuts along the eastern slope of the hillside. From here you have a breathtaking panorama of redwood-forested ridges rippling toward the coast, and on clear days, you can see Monterey Bay to the south.

You meet the broad Hickory Oaks Trail and continue straight, past your return route to Ward Road. The trail meanders up, over, down, and around oak-topped grassy knolls. You come to a short detour on a small singletrack, which affords great views west and south. On the main trail again, you descend a wide, rocky section to reach Skyline Blvd.

Turn around at Skyline Blvd. and retrace your steps to the junction on the Hickory Oaks Trail and turn left to take the alternate return route to Ward Road. The wide trail descends open, grassy slopes pocketed by dark clusters of bay laurel and oak. You pass junctions with the Ranch Spring Trail and School Road. Watch for deteriorated pavement that crops up beneath the dirt along this section of Ward Road. Hazelnut and wild rose line the trail, and oak, bay laurel, and buckeye offer shade as it curves in and out of ravines.

After a steady climb back to the ridge you join Long Ridge Road and continue straight (north). Gentle ups and downs on open grasslands define the ridgetop trail, and dramatic coastal views stretch northward. You veer right on the Long Ridge Trail, now a single-track, and pass through a wooden gate that bars bikes and horses. The cool, shaded trail descends gently on switchbacks into a mixed forest of oak, bay laurel, Douglas-fir, and madrone; leaf duff covers rocks and roots in the path. Stay on the Long Ridge Trail past a junction with a spur to the Peters Creek Trail. After a short switchback climb, the trail leads briefly through chaparral, where manzanita and chamise grow in the dry, rocky soil.

Watch for fallen twigs littering the trail. Private Portola Heights Road is on your left and a path leading to it crosses your trail. When sunlight strikes the tall madrone trees that grow here, a reddish-gold cast hangs over the forest. Now you begin to descend increasingly steep switchbacks to the floor of Peters Creek Canyon. Turn left on the Peters Creek Trail and retrace your steps 0.5 mile to the trailhead.

Alternate Routes

Long Ridge Preserve offers plenty of options for shorter runs; one is to skip the Hickory Oaks segment of the featured run. Coastal views are a major highlight of this preserve, so a stint along the ridgetop is recommended. For longer runs, explore the Bay Area Ridge Trail route north toward Skyline Preserve or south toward Saratoga Gap. You can link to Monte Bello Preserve via the Grizzly Flat Trail (Run 39), which begins just across Skyline Blvd. from the Long Ridge trailhead.

Trail Notes

- Singletracks and old ranch roads
- Narrow in spots; some root and rock obstacles; some muddy patches after wet weather
- Dog permit required for first 0.4 mile; no dogs allowed beyond (dogs and their companions can head north along the Bay Area Ridge Trail)
- Bikes allowed
- Horses allowed
- No toilet or water
- No fees
- Auto noise along Skyline Blvd. is nearly constant at Long Ridge

Nature Notes

Hickory oak is another name for the tree commonly known as canyon oak, and has the hardest wood of all western oaks. It also is the most widely distributed oak in California and lives in a variety of habitats and plant communities. The trees grow on hillsides and ridges and in canyons from Oregon to Baja California, between sea level and 9000 feet. Although individual trees vary in form and characteristics, all canyon oaks have distinctive holly-like leaves with shiny upper surfaces and pale blue or greyish undersides, often covered with soft felt-like hairs. Their acorns are 1–2 inches long, with thick cups that are covered with smooth felt hairs.

 See Russian Ridge (Run 42) for suggestions.

41

BLACK MOUNTAIN LOOP AT MONTE BELLO

The smooth slopes of Monte Bello Ridge rise from Stevens Creek Canyon, where the San Andreas fault cuts through the Santa Cruz Mountains. Cross grassy hillsides pocketed with buckeyes and deciduous oaks, detour to Black Mountain for views of the Diablo Range, and descend chaparral slopes into a bay laurel-shaded canyon. You'll climb gradually on exposed singletrack trails, descend steeply on a wide, gravelly trail, and make some short, stiff ascents as you return to the trailhead.

Distance	4.4 miles
Time	0.5-1 hour
Type	semi-loop
High Point/Low Point	2690′/1909′
Difficulty	moderate
Use	moderate
Maps	MROSD map at trailhead
Area Management	Midpeninsula Regional Open Space District

From Palo Alto, take Page Mill Rd. 7 miles west from Hwy. 280 (1 mile east from Skyline Blvd.) to the Monte Bello main parking area. From Skyline Blvd, turn east on Page Mill Rd. and go 1 mile to the parking area.

Trailhead Access

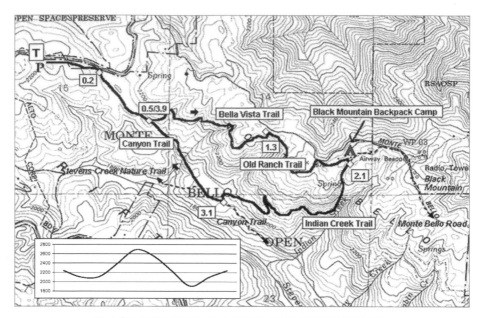

BLACK MOUNTAIN LOOP AT MONTE BELLO

Route Directions

Begin on roadside singletrack and follow to MB03 trailhead.

0.2 Turn right on **Canyon Trail**.

0.5 Turn left on **Bella Vista Trail**.

1.3 Veer right on **Old Ranch Trail**.

1.8 Follow gravel road to Backpack Camp.

1.9 Turn right on **Indian Creek Trail** at Backpack Camp.

2.0 Turn left on wide dirt trail.

2.1 Turn right sharply to continue on Indian Creek Trail.

3.1 Turn right on **Canyon Trail**.

3.3 Pass Stevens Creek Nature Trail.

3.9 Pass Bella Vista Trail.

About the Trail

Leave the main parking area on a small trail that borders Page Mill Road; after 0.2 mile, you reach MB03 gate (fewer parking spots and no bathrooms) and the beginning of the Canyon Trail. You descend gradually on the wide, smooth trail, bordered by blackberry, coyote bush, and willows. Shortly, you turn left on the singletrack Bella Vista Trail and cross a broad grassy slope on a gentle uphill grade. Below you lies the tree-filled cavity of Stevens Creek Canyon, where the Canyon Trail follows the creek. Your smooth trail winds in and out of ravines where small creekbeds descend the hillside and grand decid-uous oaks drop their leaves in fall and winter. In spring, pink-tinged new growth sprouts from the old branches. As you gain elevation and round a high knoll, your views extend west across the ridges of the Santa Cruz Mountains toward the coast, and ahead of you to Black Mountain.

The gravel Monte Bello Road parallels your trail intermittently on its route to Black Mountain. You leave the Bella Vista Trail and join the singletrack Old Ranch Trail. Looking toward the coast, you see in the foreground the Christmas Tree Farm at Skyline Ridge Open Space Preserve, where orderly lines of planted fir trees stand out among the natural irregularity of oaks, redwoods, and bay laurel. The trail continues to climb toward Black Mountain; a cluster of buckeye fills a ravine, the branches bare and dramatic in fall and win-ter, and covered with fragrant flower spikes in spring. Your views broaden and extend to Mt. Diablo, the Diablo Range across the South Bay, and to Mt. Umunhum and Loma Prieta Mountain in the Santa Cruz Mountain Range.

After almost 2 miles from the trailhead you reach the Black Mountain Backpack Camp, where you'll find toilets, nonpotable water, and a phone. You branch right here on a singletrack that cuts across the hillside to a wide dirt trail. Go left and soon meet the Indian Creek Trail. To detour to the top of Black Mountain (0.8 mile round trip and incredible views), turn left at the junction with the Indian Creek Trail. Otherwise, turn right and descend the wide, exposed trail into Stevens Creek Canyon. The continuous downhill grade alternates between moderate and steep as it crosses chaparral- and grass-covered hillsides. As you near the Canyon Trail at the bot-tom, the slopes become more wooded; the moss-covered branches of an enormous oak stretch across the trail.

Turn right on the Canyon Trail, where you immediately begin to climb on a wide, duff-covered trail beneath bay laurel, oak, and Douglas-fir. High above Stevens Creek, you emerge at the base of the exposed slopes of Black Mountain; across the canyon, dense red-woods cover the hillside. A steep uphill lies between you and the trailhead, but it is at least a shaded climb.

Alternate Routes

The Canyon Trail is one of the best trails around—an 8.6-mile out and back from Monte Bello Open Space Preserve to Stevens Canyon Road, with a few side trails along that offer loop trips. The trail follows the deep slice of the San Andreas fault through Stevens Creek Canyon. You'll pass a fault-formed sag pond, go through a lush bay-laurel forest, and occasionally pass beneath the steep grassy slopes that rise to Black Mountain.

Trail Notes
- Singletrack trails and old ranch roads
- Canyon Trail rocky in parts; Indian Creek Trail steep downhill
- No dogs
- Bikes allowed
- Horses allowed
- Toilet at trailhead and Black Mountain Backpack Camp
- No water
- No fees
- Canyon Trail is popular with mountain bikers

You won't find many food options close to this preserve. Instead, bring some snacks or a picnic lunch. A stone bench on the Stevens Creek Nature Trail is a great place to replenish your energy; views from the bench look south over Stevens Creek Canyon to Mt. Umunhum and Loma Prieta, and west toward the Pacific. To get there, take the Stevens Creek Nature Trail for about 0.1 mile from the parking area.

Nature Notes
From the northern boundary of Monte Bello Preserve, you can trace the wide trough of the San Andreas fault as it cuts through Stevens Creek Canyon and extends south through the Santa Cruz Mountains to Mt. Umunhum and Loma Prieta Mountain. (Loma Prieta was the epicenter of the 7.1 magnitude earthquake that shook the Bay Area in 1989.) When the San Andreas moves, the two plates on either side of it (the North American and the Pacific) slide past each other horizontally in what is called a "strike/slip" movement. Sag ponds often form along strike/slip faults because this movement creates depressions where water collects above an impermeable rock layer.

You'll see evidence of fault action as you follow the Canyon Trail's trajectory along the fault line. Look for the marshy sag pond, where cattails, reeds, and frogs live. Watch for rocks strewn along the trail, the likely results of movement along the fault.

42

RUSSIAN RIDGE

The smooth trails at Russian Ridge Preserve offer year-round treats. Carpets of wildflowers make this one of the best spring destinations in the Bay Area. In summer, fog often drifts up the ridge from the coast, cooling the exposed trails. The blonde hills of autumn contrast with evergreen oak and bay laurel, and on clear winter days, you'll have 360-degree views from Borel Hill.

Distance	4.7 miles
Time	0.5–1.25 hours
Type	semi-loop
High Point/Low Point	2562′/2246′
Difficulty	easy
Use	heavy
Maps	MROSD map at trailhead
Area Management	Midpeninsula Regional Open Space District

Take Page Mill Rd. from Palo Alto, Woodside/La Honda Rd. (Hwy. 84) from Woodside, or Hwy. 92 to Skyline Blvd. Park at the preserve parking lot at the junction of Alpine Rd. and Skyline Blvd., where Page Mill Rd. meets Skyline Blvd. from the west. **Trailhead Access**

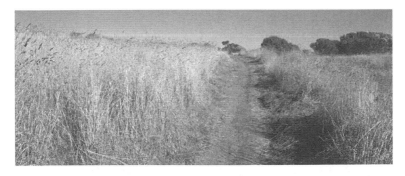

Ridge Trail

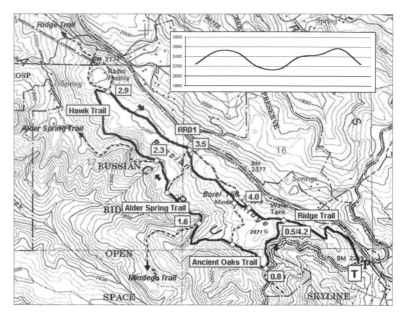

RUSSIAN RIDGE

Route Directions Begin on unsigned Ridge Trail.

0.5 Turn left on connector to Ancient Oaks Trail.

0.8 Turn right on **Ancient Oaks Trail.**

1.1 Pass connector to Ridge Trail.

1.6 Turn right on **Alder Spring Trail;** Mindego Trail goes left.

1.9 Pass connector to Ridge Trail.

2.3 Veer right on **Hawk Trail.**

2.9 Turn right on **Ridge Trail.**

3.5 Pass connector to Alder Spring Trail. Just beyond, veer right on singletrack trail.

3.9 Pass connector to Ancient Oaks Trail.

4.0 Rejoin **Ridge Trail.**

4.2 Pass connector to Ancient Oaks Trail.

About the Trail This route begins east of the ridge and makes a short, gentle climb on the wide Ridge Trail (also part of the Bay Area Ridge Trail). A stand of buckeye graces the grassy slope that rises to your left. At the ridgetop, you have a sweeping view of the coast, often laced with fog.

You leave the Ridge Trail here on a connector to the Ancient Oaks Trail and descend gradually west. The trail passes large oak and bay laurel trees on the exposed hillside, high above Alpine Road. On clear days you'll see Monterey Bay in the distance, beyond the lofty ridges of the Santa Cruz Mountains.

The Ancient Oaks Trail heads north on a level course across grassy slopes. In spring these vibrant, green hillsides shine with poppies, lupine, goldfields, and checkerbloom; in fall the grasses turn brittle and golden. Your view takes in Pescadero's broad valley, located beyond a series of westward-rolling ridges. In the foreground, you see volcanic Mindego Hill and the wide Mindego Trail winding toward it.

The Ancient Oaks Trail leaves the open slopes and descends slightly into an exceptional forested area for which the trail is named. The knotted, moss-covered oak trunks here are enormous in girth, and their curved branches spread out hundreds of feet. These graceful oaks are canyon oaks—notice their characteristically large acorns beneath your feet.

You turn right on the Alder Spring Trail and head into grasslands again. Open slopes rise steeply east to the ridge. A connector trail to the Ridge Trail branches right (taking it is a good way to shorten this route), but you continue on the Alder Spring Trail. Oak and bay laurel line the ravine of Mindego Creek, which descends the hillside from the east and crosses beneath the trail.

You eventually return to the ridgetop on the Hawk Trail, a singletrack that angles up a grassy slope on a gradual climb. Pass a small trail that goes left to climb the low knoll, and head right (south), passing large stands of coyote bush that have taken hold on these hillsides. At the next junction, go right on the Ridge Trail to begin your ridgetop return to the trailhead. On this broad trail, you can see east across the bay to the Diablo Range, and west to the coast.

After passing a connector to the Alder Spring Trail, branch left on the small singletrack that wraps around a low slope of Borel Hill and offers great views of the coast. In spring, you'll whisk through thigh-high grasses that line this narrow trail. Just beyond the summit of 2572-foot Borel Hill, you rejoin the wide Ridge Trail. (Detour to the top of the hill for 360-degree views of the bay, coast, and mountains.) Return to the trailhead on a gentle descent.

Alternate Routes The connecting trails between the Ridge Trail and the Ancient Oaks and Alder Springs trails offer plenty of opportunities to shorten this route. For a longer run, cross to the east side of Skyline Blvd. at RR01 (where the Ridge Trail and the connector to Alder Springs Trail meet) and explore the trails in Coal Creek Open Space Preserve (Run 43).

Trail Notes
- Singletrack and fire trails
- Mostly smooth trails; Hawk Trail rutted
- No dogs
- Bikes allowed
- Horses allowed
- Toilet at trailhead; no water
- No fees

 The pickings are slim along this section of Skyline Blvd. For the most variety, head down Page Mill Road into Palo Alto; other options are Alice's Restaurant and the grocery store at the intersection of Skyline Blvd. and Hwy. 84.

Nature Notes
 Russian Ridge Preserve is often cited as one of the top five places to see spring wildflowers in the Bay Area. Visit the preserve then to admire abundant poppies, lupine, mule ears, clarkia, and blue dicks. You may see some wildlife here too—the preserve is one of the Bay Area's best places to watch raptors. Hawks, turkey vultures, and golden eagles soar overhead on strong updrafts, searching for smaller birds, snakes, and rodents to prey on—and carrion, in the case of the vultures. Coyotes and an occasional mountain lion roam the ridges and the protected canyons.

43

COAL CREEK FIGURE 8

This short figure-8 loop is one of the few trails on the peninsula where dogs are allowed, and it offers longer or shorter options aplenty. Coal Creek is sheltered when Skyline ridge is windy or cloaked in fog, and cool when the sun heats up routes on the exposed ridge. Mostly wide and shaded trails compose this loop, with one stiff, exposed uphill on the final leg.

Distance	4 miles
Time	0.5–1 hour
Type	double loop
High Point/Low Point	2145´/1704´
Difficulty	moderate
Use	light
Maps	MROSD map available across Skyline Blvd. from Caltrans Vista Point at Russian Ridge trailhead, gate RR01
Area Management	Midpeninsula Regional Open Space District

Trailhead Access

Take Page Mill Rd. from Palo Alto, Woodside/La Honda Rd. (Hwy. 84) from Woodside, or Hwy. 92 to Skyline Blvd. Park at the Caltrans Vista Point on the east side of the road, 8.9 miles south of Hwy. 84 and 1.2 miles north of Page Mill Rd. Russian Ridge Trailhead RR01 is directly across the road.

Coal Creek is also accessible from Page Mill Rd.: park in the Monte Bello parking lot, 8.0 miles west of Interstate 280, and go west on the trail that parallels the road to MB05 gate. Cross Page Mill to the gated, unsigned Alpine Rd.

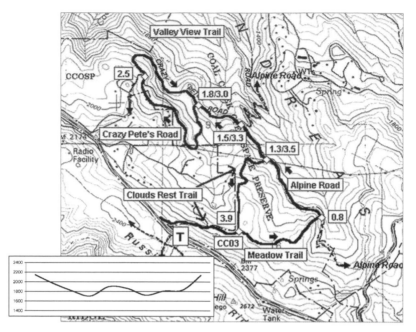

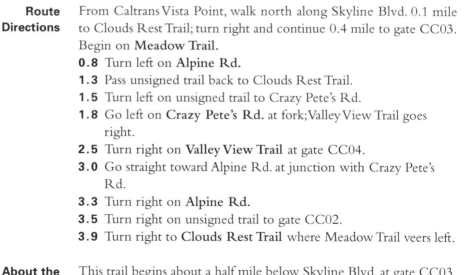

COAL CREEK FIGURE 8

Route Directions

From Caltrans Vista Point, walk north along Skyline Blvd. 0.1 mile to Clouds Rest Trail; turn right and continue 0.4 mile to gate CC03. Begin on **Meadow Trail.**

0.8 Turn left on **Alpine Rd.**

1.3 Pass unsigned trail back to Clouds Rest Trail.

1.5 Turn left on unsigned trail to Crazy Pete's Rd.

1.8 Go left on **Crazy Pete's Rd.** at fork; Valley View Trail goes right.

2.5 Turn right on **Valley View Trail** at gate CC04.

3.0 Go straight toward Alpine Rd. at junction with Crazy Pete's Rd.

3.3 Turn right on **Alpine Rd.**

3.5 Turn right on unsigned trail to gate CC02.

3.9 Turn right to **Clouds Rest Trail** where Meadow Trail veers left.

About the Trail

This trail begins about a half mile below Skyline Blvd. at gate CC03. Take in the view from the Caltrans Vista Point and then head north along the shoulder of Skyline Blvd. for about 0.1 mile. Turn right on

Clouds Rest Trail, marked with a green street sign, and descend steeply on this paved road to a large house and gate CC03 —the beginning of the Meadow Trail.

The Meadow Trail is at first a wide, fairly level road shaded by oak and bay laurel. You quickly come to an open meadow with views across the Santa Clara Valley to the Diablo Range. In spring, bright California poppies, lupine, and checkerbloom intermingle with grasses and coyote bush. Bear right on the Meadow Trail to begin the first loop. Beyond a small rise mossy oaks arch overhead and their leaves pad the soft dirt path. The trail descends through this shaded patch of oak and bay laurel and emerges to another open meadow, with more views and more spring wildflowers. Across the meadow, you continue your gentle descent to Alpine Road through oak and madrone.

Follow Alpine Road gradually downhill, high above a deep creekbed shaded by deciduous oaks and bay laurel. The wide road's dirt- and gravel-surface keeps it mud-free even in wet weather, and colorful oak leaves cover it in fall and winter. Blackberry, ferns, coyote bush, and mountain mahogany grow on the trail's banks.

Continue past the first left-branching singletrack (the return route to the Meadow Trail). After 0.2 you reach another unsigned, left-branching trail. Follow this narrow path (Crazy Pete's Road) to a small stream, where water cascades down the steep hillside in the rainy season. Big-leaf maple and creek dogwood border the stream, the bare red twigs of the dogwood colorful in winter. Cross the wooden bridge and continue past a thicket of thimbleberry to the junction with the Valley View Trail. Stay left on Crazy Pete's Road, now a wide trail that climbs under the cover of oak and bay laurel. Loop back on the Valley View Trail by turning right at the next junction. Descend gradually past large madrone, taking in vistas true to the trail's name.

From the junction with Crazy Pete's Road, retrace your steps to Alpine Road and turn right. To complete the figure-8 loop, take the next right-branching trail, the Clouds Rest Trail, and cross through gate CC02. Climb steeply to a broad, grassy plateau; in spring, lupine and poppies bloom among the grasses. A power tower looms above, and you have a clear view of the ridge ahead. After a brief, level break you continue climbing the sandy trail, enjoying far-reaching views east. About a half mile from Alpine Road, you reach the

Meadow Trail, where you began the loop, and turn right to shortly return to the trailhead.

Alternate Routes One of the best features of this run is the number of additional route options available. Extend this route by crossing Skyline Blvd. into Russian Ridge Open Space Preserve; go left on the Borel Hill Trail and continue along the ridgetop for fabulous coastal views. Or do the loop described in Russian Ridge (Run 42). To link to trails in Monte Bello Open Space Preserve, turn right from the Meadow Trail onto Alpine Road, and continue 0.5 mile to Page Mill Road. Cross the road and follow a short trail to gate MB04 to enter the preserve.

Or to shorten the featured route, just run one loop.

Trail Notes
- Singletrack and fire trails
- Smooth trails; leaf duff; some mud on Meadow Trail in rainy season
- Dogs on leash
- Bikes allowed
- Horses allowed
- No toilet or water
- No fees

 See Russian Ridge (Run 42) for suggestions.

44

HAMMS GULCH LOOP

A gradual climb on a shaded path takes you from Portola Valley to Skyline ridge in Windy Hill Open Space Preserve. You'll have views of the coast and the bay from the ridge, and then descend on gentle switchbacks through oak, bay, and madrone. Be warned, however, that Windy Hill lives up to its name. Winters can be chilly, but most of the year you'll appreciate the relief from the warm Santa Clara Valley temperatures.

Distance	9.8 miles
Time	1.25–2.5 hours
Type	semi-loop
High Point/Low Point	1872′/537′
Difficulty	moderate
Use	moderate
Maps	MROSD map at trailhead
Area Management	Midpeninsula Regional Open Space District

Exit I-280 at Alpine Rd. Go west on Alpine Rd. 3.0 miles to Portola Rd. Turn right and continue 0.8 mile to Windy Hill Preserve entrance on the left. **Trailhead Access**

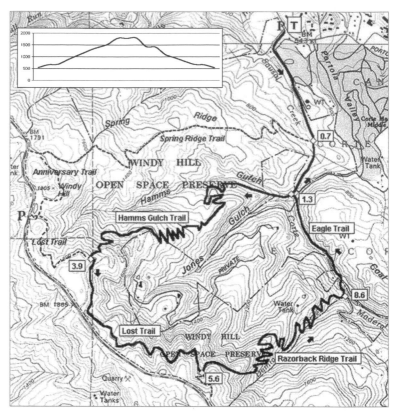

HAMMS GULCH LOOP

Route Directions

0.1 Turn left, follow signs to Spring Ridge Trail.

0.7 Pass turnoff to Spring Ridge Trail.

0.9 Pass second turnoff to Spring Ridge Trail.

1.3 Turn right on **Hamms Gulch Trail.**

3.9 Turn left on **Lost Trail.**

4.1 Cross gravel road; continue straight.

5.6 Veer left on **Razorback Ridge Trail.**

7.9 Turn left on road, follow TRAIL sign.

8.0 Cross creek on road. Turn left on paved road, then veer left on **Eagle Trail.**

8.5 Turn left and cross creek on road, following signs to Hamms Gulch Trail. Turn right and cross wooden footbridge.

8.6 Turn right where Hamms Gulch Trail goes straight, follow signs to Alpine and Portola roads. Retrace route to trailhead.

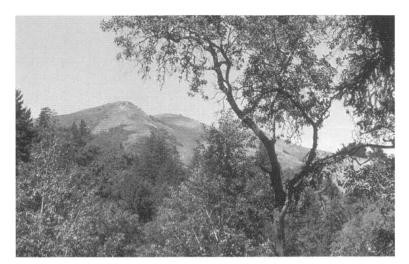

View of Windy Hill from Hamms Gulch Trail

The gravel road from the trailhead quickly becomes a wide dirt trail and passes a small pond formed by dammed Sausal Creek. Coyote bush and coffeeberry line the trail and the lofty branches of majestic black oaks stretch overhead. The open grasslands here are exposed and often hot on warm days.

Shortly you reach the Hamms Gulch Trail, which initially climbs a small hill and then continues gently toward the ridgetop on switchbacks. Big-leaf maple, madrone, buckeye, and bay laurel provide welcome shade and relief from the sun. In late summer and fall colorful leaves decorate the trail; look for hound's tongue and trillium on the forest floor in early spring. As you ascend the narrow trail, you'll catch glimpses of the grassy slopes of Windy Hill through the trees.

You emerge briefly from the shade and pass an open hillside, where abundant wildflowers bloom in spring. Thick moss covers the trunks of live oak trees as you near the ridgetop, evidence of the fog that often flows up and over the hills from the coast. The trail may be squishy with mud from the fog's moisture.

You trace the ridgetop on the Lost Trail, a splendid singletrack. In spring and summer, you'll see sticky monkeyflower, penstemon, lupine, and Indian paintbrush in bloom. Thimbleberry thrives in the filtered shade of live oak, big-leaf maple, and Douglas-fir. You wind around gullies where the trail is eroded in spots, and narrow, rutted sections keep you alert. Look behind you for glimpses of the Spring Ridge Trail (see **Alternate Routes** below) as it descends an open grassy slope.

On the shaded Razorback Ridge Trail you ease down the ridge on well-graded switchbacks. A deep ravine borders the singletrack trail, and red-barked madrone, deep-green bay laurel, and majestic oak create a collage of color and texture, especially beautiful in fall. Rampant poison oak crawls over ferns, star flower, and false solomon's seal in the understory, but it doesn't encroach on the path. Leaf duff may obscure rocks and roots, so watch your step. As you near the bottom, the trail sidles along the edge of a canyon and becomes narrow in spots.

The Razorback Ridge Trail ends at a dirt road; follow the road to cross Corte Madera Creek and meet Alpine Road. After a few steps on the pavement you join the Eagle Trail and descend to parallel the creek. You cross the creek and then shortly pass your earlier turn-off to the Hamm's Gulch Trail; from there, retrace your steps back to the trailhead.

Alternate Routes   Your dog can join you on a 7.8-mile loop at Windy Hill. Start on the Hamms Gulch Trail and turn right at the ridgetop on the Lost Trail. Join the Anniversary Trail to reach the Spring Ridge Trail, a wide, exposed fire trail with great views of the Santa Clara Valley, the bay, and the Diablo Range.

Trail Notes   • Fire trail and singletrack
• Leaf duff on Razorback Ridge Trail may obscure rocks and roots; some narrow spots
• Leashed dogs allowed on Hamms Gulch, Anniversary, and Spring Ridge trails
• Bikes allowed on Spring Ridge and upper Anniversary trails
• Horses allowed on all trails on this route; Lost, Hamms Gulch, Razorback Ridge trails closed to equestrians seasonally
• Toilet at trailhead
• No water
• No fees

 Bianchini's Market is well-stocked and conveniently located near the trailhead. You'll find it on Alpine Road, near the junction with I-280.

45

WINDY HILL RIDGELINE

This route's Lost Trail offers the best of Windy Hill Preserve: masses of spring wildflowers on open slopes; colorful big-leaf-maple leaves in fall; oak, bay laurel, and Douglas-fir among lush vegetation; and views of the Diablo Range across the bay, beyond a foreground of forested gulches and open hillsides. The trail begins on Skyline ridge at about 1800 feet and hugs the ridgeline just beneath its crest, losing and gaining little elevation.

Distance	5 miles
Time	0.75–1.25 hours
Type	out-and-back
High Point/Low Point	1997′/1787′
Difficulty	easy
Use	moderate
Maps	MROSD map at trailhead
Area Management	Midpeninsula Regional Open Space District

Trailhead Access

Take Page Mill Rd. from Palo Alto, Woodside/La Honda Rd. (Hwy. 84) from Woodside, or Hwy. 92 to Skyline Blvd. Parking lot is 2.3 miles south of Woodside/La Honda Rd., or 4.9 miles north of Page Mill Rd. on east side of Skyline Blvd.

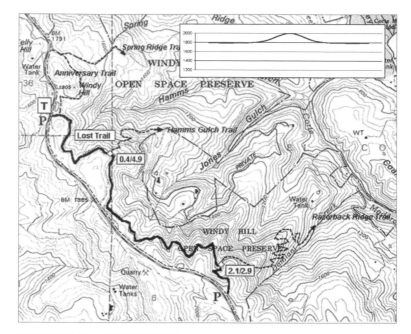

WINDY HILL RIDGELINE

Route Directions

Turn right at trailhead to begin on **Lost Trail**.
0.4 Pass Hamms Gulch Trail.
0.6 Pass offshoot to Skyline Blvd.
2.1 Pass Razorback Ridge Trail.
2.5 Skyline Blvd. Retrace route to trailhead.

About the Trail

The Lost Trail begins as a smooth singletrack, winding in and out of gullies on the east side of the ridge. Erosion threatens the trail in spots and some narrow, rutted sections and a few roots interrupt the path. After about half a mile, you cross a wide, gravel service road and continue straight on the Lost Trail, headed for the Razorback Ridge Trail.

Fog moistens the trail beneath Douglas-fir, live oak, and bay laurel, and thimbleberry and tanbark oak thrive in the understory. On exposed slopes, coyote bush, blackberry, and poison oak grow in dry, rocky soil. Across the bay, you'll see 4213-foot Mt. Hamilton, the highest point in the Bay Area. Look behind you for glimpses of 1905-foot Windy Hill, the preserve's highest point; you also can see the Spring Ridge Trail as it descends grassy slopes beyond.

Look for wildflowers along the trail as early as January—pink currant flowers and purple hound's tongue bloom first; honeysuckle, clarkia, and thimbleberry bloom throughout the spring, and as late as August, you may see lupine, Indian paintbrush, penstemon, and sticky monkeyflower.

The Lost Trail ends at Skyline Blvd., where you turn around to retrace your steps to the trailhead.

Alternate Routes

To extend this run, turn left from the main trailhead for a 1.4-mile round trip on the Anniversary Trail. This narrow singletrack skirts Windy Hill's rounded knolls and offers sweeping views of the South Bay and the coast. Wildflowers coat the open hillside in spring.

For a more challenging run, descend the Spring Ridge, Hamms Gulch, or Razorback Ridge trails (Run 44).

Trail Notes

- Singletrack trail
- Some narrow, rutted sections
- No dogs on Lost Trail; leashed dogs allowed on Hamms Gulch, Anniversary, and Spring Ridge trails
- No bikes on Lost Trail; bikes allowed on Spring Ridge and upper Anniversary trails
- Lost Trail closed to horses seasonally, as are Hamms Gulch and Razorback Ridge trails
- Toilet at trailhead
- No water
- No fees

Look for snacks at the grocery store located where Skyline Blvd. and Hwy. 84 intersect.

46

EL CORTE DE MADERA LOOP

Smooth, fast singletracks wind through lush redwood forests and top out on chaparral slopes with views of the Pacific. This preserve's trails descend the west side of Skyline ridge and offer moderate and challenging routes. Also, visit the unusual sandstone formation this preserve is known for.

Distance	7.3 miles (+1.2 round trip to sandstone formation)
Time	1-2 hours
Type	loop
High Point/Low Point	2389′/1583′
Difficulty	moderate
Use	heavy
Maps	MROSD map at trailhead
Area Management	Midpeninsula Regional Open Space District

Trailhead Access Take Page Mill Rd. from Palo Alto, Woodside/La Honda Rd. (Hwy. 84) from Woodside, or Hwy. 92 to Skyline Blvd. Park at Skeggs Point Caltrans Vista Point, 5.4 miles north of Hwy. 84 and 7.6 miles south of Hwy. 92. Trailhead is CM01 gate, across the road and 100 yards to the north.

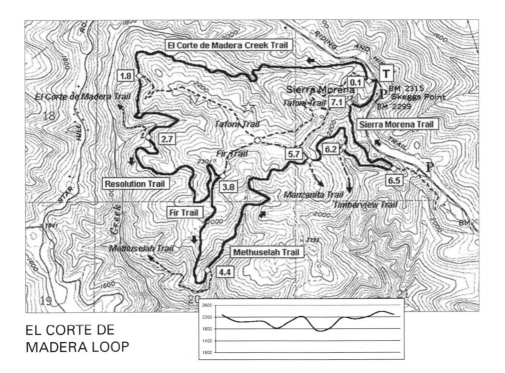

EL CORTE DE
MADERA LOOP

CM01 gate. Begin on **Tafoni Trail.**

0.1 Turn right on **El Corte de Madera Creek Trail.**

0.8 Turn left on wooden bridge, following El Corte de Madera Creek Trail.

1.8 Pass turnoff to Tafoni Trail.

2.7 Turn left on **Resolution Trail.**

3.8 Turn right on **Fir Trail.**

4.4 Turn left on **Methuselah Trail.**

5.7 Continue straight on Methuselah Trail at junction with Manzanita and Fir trails.

6.2 Turn left on **Methuselah Trail** at junction with Timberview Trail.

6.5 Turn left on **Sierra Morena Trail.**

7.1 Turn right on **Fir Trail.** Follow paved road 0.2 mile to CM01.

Route Directions

For 1.2 mile round trip detour to sandstone formation:

- Turn left (northeast) on **Fir Trail.**
- Make a sharp left on **Tafoni Trail.**
- Turn right on side trail to sandstone formation
- Retrace steps to Fir Trail.

About the Trail

Begin at the CM01 MROSD gate and briefly join the Tafoni Trail, your link to the El Corte de Madera Creek Trail. Climb gently on the shaded trail to the first junction. Turn right on the wide El Corte de Madera Creek Trail and descend into a deep canyon of lush redwoods. Mossy rocks lie in the creekbed and tanbark oak, honey-suckle, blackberry, and bunchgrasseses cover the hillsides. Watch for roots and rocks.

Towering redwoods dwarf you in this deep canyon, and tall bunchgrasses and ferns grow close to the creek. The moist forest accents the fragrance of bay laurel and redwood. Redwood needles coat the trail, joined by big-leaf maple leaves in fall. Your descent is mostly gentle, sometimes moderate, but always well graded.

You cross a wooden bridge and the trail becomes a singletrack lined by abundant tanbark oak and ferns. After a moderate climb it hugs the hillside on a fairly level course; gentle uphills gradually take you higher and higher on the side of the deep redwood canyon. The forest composition changes here as more sunlight penetrates the tree cover, now dominated by oaks rather than redwoods. Tanbark oaks and huckleberry grow abundantly beneath higher branches, and high ferns and thick stands of bunchgrass line the fast trail in spots.

The trail's sandy dirt is evidence of the sandstone that this preserve is known for. In wet weather, muddy puddles gather in depressions along this singletrack, but they are only a minor obstacle. Other obstacles are the roots and rocks that lurk beneath the duff, the occasional downed tree that blocks the trail, and the mountain bikers who also love these singletrack trails. When you hear a biker coming, step to the side as soon as you can; many bikers will pull over for you as well.

The trail proceeds to hug the hillside above a deep canyon, winding in and out of gullies until it reaches a junction with the Resolution Trail. You climb out of the redwoods on the exposed Resolution Trail into chaparral, where thick manzanita and abundant madrone dominate the rocky soil. The air is warmer and fragrant, and you have views west across the sea of redwoods that stretches to the coast. You dip in and out of redwoods and chaparral, gently ascending and descending.

On the Fir Trail, you return to the deep canyon (unless you choose to visit the Tafoni Sandstone or return to the trailhead by turning left on the Fir Trail). Instead of redwoods, Douglas-firs and chaparral—madrone, manzanita, and coffeeberry—cover the drier slopes. The trail is rocky and steep and may be slippery in sections. You'll have incredible views of the Santa Cruz Mountains as they ripple toward the coast.

Regain your lost elevation on the Methuselah Trail—a wide, shaded logging road that winds through redwood, Douglas-fir, and tanbark oak—which climbs moderately to the ridge. A level stretch about a mile from the ridgetop gives you a break before one last uphill stint. As you round the last bend, you see and hear cars along Skyline Blvd.

The Methuselah Trail ends at the CM02 gate, but you veer left on the Sierra Morena Trail to return to Skeggs Point. The smooth dirt singletrack heads north just below Skyline Blvd.; it meets the Fir Trail and passes a toilet and a power station, and continues on a paved road to the CM01 gate and the end of this loop.

Alternate Routes

For an easier 5-mile loop, skip the stiff uphill on the Methuselah Trail and return to the trailhead on the Fir or Tafoni trails.

Trail Notes

- Singletrack and fire trails
- Narrow in spots; some root and rock obstacles; steep and slippery sections on Fir Trail to Methuselah Trail
- No dogs
- Bikes allowed
- Horses allowed
- Toilet at Skeggs Point parking area; no water
- No fees
- Popular with mountain bikers

See Skyline Trail: Huddart to Wunderlich (Run 48) for suggestions.

Nature Notes

Sandstone is an important geological component of the Santa Cruz Mountains and is largely responsible for the delightfully soft and smooth trails that crisscross the mountains' parks and preserves. Along some trails, you'll notice large sandstone formations marked by deep caves and pockets; some also have an intriguing honeycomb configuration on their surface. These unique shapes, called tafoni, are created by a complicated weathering process. Sandstone is composed of large-grained sand particles, cemented together by calcium carbonate. During California's cool, wet winters, rainwater penetrates the rock crevices and slowly dissolves the calcium carbonate, breaking down its adhesive quality and slowly eroding the sandstone. The warm and dry weather typical of California's long summers draws the calcium carbonate to the rocks' surface and forms a hard, weather-resistant crust. A cavity then forms beneath the outer layer. Over time, the crust collapses and exposes the sculptured formations in the pocket.

The large sandstone formation in El Corte de Madera is an unexpected outcropping that juts some 50 feet into the air beneath a thick tree cover.

WUNDERLICH COUNTY PARK

Wunderlich County Park covers nearly 1,000 acres on the eastern slope of the Santa Cruz Mountains, extending from the town of Woodside to Skyline ridge. Second-growth redwoods and mixed evergreen forests of oak and madrone swathe the hillsides; open meadows, sprinkled with wildflowers in spring, allow views across the South Bay.

The park has 25 miles of well-signed, well-graded trails that offer short, easy loops and longer, steeper routes. From "The Crossroads," the Skyline Trail climbs to the ridge and then continues along its crest for about 5 miles (also the Bay Area Ridge Trail) to Huddart Park (Run 48).

In fall, the chilly air triggers the change in leaf color on the bay laurels, big-leaf maples, buckeyes, and poison oak; the green forest flushes with muted reds and golds. Most of Wunderlich's trails are shaded, so the park is also a good bet in summer; in winter, rains make many trails muddy.

What You'll Find

Wunderlich County Park is open from 8 AM to dark. Dogs and bikes are not allowed on trails, but horses are. Toilets and water are at the trailhead. You'll also find a signpost that stocks maps.

47

LOOP TRIP TO
SKYLINE RIDGE

Choose between a double and a single loop on Wunderlich's smooth trails, under the cover of redwoods, oak, bay laurel, and madrone. From open meadows, you'll have views of the Diablo Range across the bay, and as you near Skyline ridge, the scent and feel of fog often waft up from the coast.

Distance	4.7 or 10.1 miles
Time	0.5–2.5 hours
Type	loop
High Point/Low Point	2234´/481´
Difficulty	moderate-strenuous
Use	moderate
Maps	park map at trailhead
Area Management	San Mateo County

Trailhead Access From I-280 in Woodside, take the Woodside Rd. exit (Hwy. 84) and head west on Woodside Rd. for 2.5 miles. Turn right into the Wunderlich County Park parking lot.

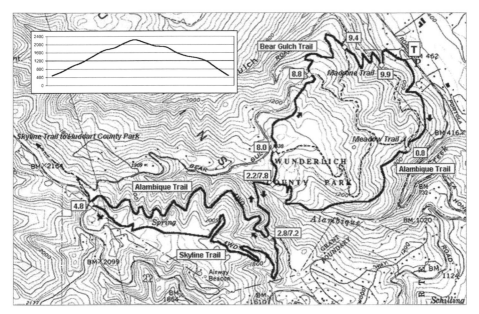

LOOP TRIP TO SKYLINE RIDGE

Begin on paved service road from parking lot.

Veer left on **Alambique Trail.**

0.7 Pass Loop Trail.

0.8 Pass Meadow Trail.

1.9 Stay right at Alambique Flat.

2.0 Pass Oak Trail.

2.2 Bear Gulch Trail.

Single loop: Turn right here and return to trailhead on Bear Gulch Trail.

Double loop: Continue on Alambique Trail.

2.8 Veer right at the Crossroads; stay on Alambique Trail.

4.8 Turn left on **Skyline Trail** at Skyline Blvd.

7.2 Rejoin **Alambique Trail** at the Crossroads.

7.8 Veer left on **Bear Gulch Trail.**

8.0 Continue straight on Bear Gulch Trail at the Meadows. Pass Meadow Trail.

8.8 Pass Redwood Flat and trail to Salamander Flat.

9.4 Pass Madrone Trail.

9.9 Pass Loop Trail.

Route Directions

About the Trail

You begin on the Alambique Trail, a wide, smooth dirt path. The well-graded trail climbs mostly gently, with some moderate sections. Through the sparse forest, you'll catch glimpses of the valley below, of the ridgeline of the Santa Cruz Mountains extending to the south, and of the mountains of the Diablo Range across the bay. Black and coast live oak, bay laurel, madrone, and buckeye shade the trail, intermittently joined by big-leaf maple, redwood, and eucalyptus. Hazelnut, ferns, and blackberry grow underneath, and poison oak creeps alongside, sometimes hanging low from tree branches.

Turn right at the junction with the Bear Gulch Trail to do the single loop. The double loop route continues on the Alambique Trail, where you are high above deep redwood canyons. You may see deer bounding through the ferns, thimbleberry, and tanbark oak that grow beneath towering redwoods and bay laurel. Views through the trees improve as you climb. You pass a large junction called The Crossroads, which you will meet again on your return route. As you draw closer to the ridgetop, you'll smell the moisture from the fog that often creeps up the western slopes to the ridgetop, dampening the trail and the lush vegetation. You pass beneath a buzzing power-line and tower, and the trail levels and reaches Skyline Blvd.

The Skyline Trail follows the ridgetop briefly, climbing gently beneath redwoods, and then descends through a thicket of scotch broom to an open patch above stables and a horse ring. A dry section of chaparral interrupts the redwood and bay-laurel forest, and tall manzanitas with mossy branches line the trail. Back in the trees, sunlight filters through the leaves and creates delicate patterns beneath your feet. A few rocks and roots are scattered under the leaf duff on the Skyline Trail, so watch your step. Otherwise, the wide, smooth trail makes for easy running, and the grade is gentle, tempered by long switchbacks.

You return to The Crossroads and retrace your steps to the Bear Gulch Trail. Veer left on this singletrack and ascend slightly on smooth dirt through drier terrain to The Meadows. Coyote bush has overtaken grasses in this open expanse, which provides the best views in the park of the lowlands of the Santa Clara Valley, the bay, and beyond to the Diablo Range.

Follow the Bear Gulch Trail back to the trailhead on a well-graded descent with some switchbacks. Oak, bay laurel, and redwood keep you cool, and in spring, prolific Douglas iris adorn the trail.

Wunderlich Park offers an array of shorter and longer routes. One shorter option begins on the Alambique Trail, turns right on the Meadow Trail, and returns via the Madrone and Bear Gulch trails to make a 2.8-mile loop. For longer runs, from Skyline Blvd. turn right to go north on the Skyline/Bay Area Ridge Trail toward Huddart County Park. Plan a shuttle trip (5.3 miles from Wunderlich to Huddart) or retrace your steps to the Wunderlich trailhead.

Alternate Routes

- Singletrack and fire trails
- Watch for roots on Skyline and Bear Gulch trails
- No dogs
- No bikes
- Horses allowed
- Toilet and water at trailhead
- No fees

Trail Notes

You'll find plenty of good food in Woodside, en route to or from I-280, just about a mile from Wunderlich. Sit down for a meal at the Woodside Bakery and Café (lunch and dinner), or Bucks Restaurant (both at the junction of Cañada and Mountain Home roads). Or try the gourmet foods at Robert's Market just across the road.

48

SKYLINE TRAIL:
HUDDART TO WUNDERLICH

This smooth singletrack hugs the east slope of Skyline ridge, winding in and out of gullies as it makes its way south. Mostly shaded by a second-growth redwood forest, it is a cool respite on warm days. Easterly views sneak through the trees. This makes a good car-shuttle run if you don't want to do the full 11+ miles, especially since the start and end points are convenient to each other.

Distance	5.8 miles one way; up to 11.6 miles
Time	up to 3 hours
Type	out-and-back or car shuttle
High Point/Low Point	2359'/1903'
Difficulty	moderate
Use	light
Maps	no map at trailhead
Area Management	San Mateo County Parks and Recreation

Trailhead Access

Northern Trailhead: Take Page Mill Rd. from Palo Alto, Woodside/La Honda Rd. (Hwy. 84) from Woodside, or Hwy. 92 to Skyline Blvd. Park at Purisima Creek Redwoods Open Space Preserve, 6.5 miles north of Hwy. 84 and 6.5 miles south of Hwy. 92. Walk across Skyline Blvd. and head north a few hundred feet to the trailhead, marked by a Bay Area Ridge Trail and Huddart Park sign.

Southern Trailhead: Take Page Mill Rd. from Palo Alto, Woodside/La Honda Rd. (Hwy. 84) from Woodside, or Hwy. 92 to Skyline Blvd. Park on the west side of the road (just south of private Bear Gulch Rd.), 3 miles north of Hwy. 84 and 10 miles south of Hwy. 92. Cross Skyline Blvd. to the trailhead in Wunderlich Park.

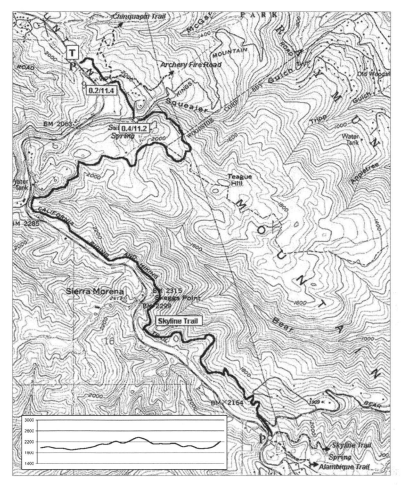

SKYLINE TRAIL: HUDDART TO WUNDERLICH

Cross Skyline Blvd. just north of the Purisima Creek parking.
Turn right at **Bay Area Ridge Trail** and Huddart Park sign.

0.1 Turn left at first junction to continue on **Skyline Trail.**

0.2 Turn right to continue on Skyline Trail.

0.4 Cross Kings Mountain Rd. and follow roadside path. Veer right and follow Bay Area Ridge Trail signs.

5.8 Wunderlich Park

NOTE: The mileage signs at either end of this trip conflict with each other. The sign in Huddart Park says 5.2 miles to Wunderlich Park; in Wunderlich, a sign says 5.7 miles to Huddart.

Route Directions

About the Trail

You begin in Huddart Park on a wide, smooth dirt road in a forest of redwood accompanied by tanbark oak, madrone, and oak. Pine-needle duff and acorns cover the trail. Depending on the day, sunlight or fog filters through the trees.

The Skyline Trail soon leaves Huddart Park and begins its southward trek along the ridge. You veer right on the singletrack and descend past a huge Douglas-fir tree to reach a private driveway that leads to Kings Mountain Road. Cross the road and briefly run parallel to it; then follow the trail into a forest of redwood and Douglas-fir. A creek descends a gully next to the road. You climb gently on the smooth, shaded trail, and emerge onto drier slopes where manzanita and chamise line the trail. In spring, large clusters of iris bloom along the trail.

You quickly return to the forest and enjoy shady cover the rest of the route. Tanbark oak, hazelnut, and huckleberry bushes grow beneath the tree cover. In fall you'll catch whiffs of bay laurel and enjoy the colorful leaves of big-leaf maple. Lanky madrones reach for light among the branches of dense redwoods. You follow the gentle swells of this smooth and delightful trail as it traces the ridgeline south toward Wunderlich Park.

Wooden posts mark off the miles as you go. After mile 5, you descend a short switchback, passing a large new house, and then climb a switchback to private Bear Gulch Road. Cross the paved road and veer right. Pick up the trail again on the left, following Bay Area Ridge Trail signs. You continue to climb on switchbacks and very soon reach the trailhead in Wunderlich Park.

Descend into Wunderlich if you like, or return to your starting point.

Alternate Routes

The trails in Huddart and Wunderlich parks that descend from the ridge are good ways to extend or vary this run. The Chinquapin Trail and Archery Fire Road head into Huddart Park just 0.2 mile from the trailhead, and connect to the park's network of trails. At the south end of this route, the Skyline Trail descends into Wunderlich Park and hooks up with the Alambique and Bear Gulch trails (Run 47), among others.

Trail Notes
- Singletrack trails
- Few obstacles
- No dogs

- No bikes
- Horses allowed
- Toilet at Purisima Creek parking
- No water
- No fees

Kings Mountain Store, just north of the northern entrance to Purisima Creek Redwoods, has a meager assortment of drinks, fruit, snacks, and deli food, plus an array of energy bars.

History Notes

Extensive redwood forests once covered the eastern slope of the Santa Cruz Mountains. In the mid-1800s logging decimated the forests; now all that remain of these ancient immense trees—some of which were over 2,000 years old—are the moss-covered stumps you pass along the trail.

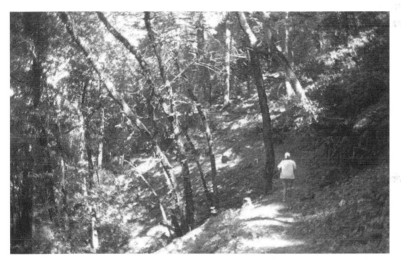

Skyline Trail

SAN PEDRO VALLEY COUNTY PARK

The 1295-acre San Pedro Valley County Park encompasses the narrow valley of San Pedro Creek and the steep slopes of Montara Mountain, where another fork of the creek descends. The 1898-foot granite bulk of Montara Mountain is the park's dominant feature, but trails also run through the valley and up and down the gentler Pacifica foothills.

San Pedro Valley Park is tucked between residential neighborhoods and San Francisco Watershed land. Although you may hear lawnmowers and children's voices as you run along these trails, you're also likely to hear or see some of the park's abundant wildlife, such as hawks, quail, garter snakes, rabbits, deer, and bobcats. In winter, steelhead salmon spawn in the two forks of San Pedro Creek that run through the park.

What You'll Find Fog and plenty of it, particularly during summer months. Although you may welcome the cool air as you climb, the fog can make for a cold and windy run. Come prepared.

Dogs are not allowed in San Pedro Valley Park. Bikes are allowed only on Weiler Ranch Road and in paved areas. Horses are allowed on some park trails—check the featured route for details. The visitor center, open weekends from 10 AM to 4 PM, provides maps and natural history information. There is a $4 parking fee. The park is open year-round from 8 AM to sunset.

49

MONTARA MOUNTAIN

Don't be scared off by the elevation gain on this run: numerous switchbacks temper the incline on the way up and preserve your knees on the descent. Impressive granite slabs, 360-degree views of the Bay Area from North Peak, and diverse native flora are the high points of this run. And the way back is all downhill!

Distance	6.4 miles
Time	0.75-1.5 hours
Type	semi-loop or out-and-back
High Point/Low Point	1898′/210′
Difficulty	moderate
Use	moderate
Maps	map at visitor center and information board
Area Management	San Pedro Valley County Park

From Hwy. 1 in Pacifica, head east on Linda Mar Blvd. After 1.6 miles, turn right on Oddstad Blvd. Turn left immediately into the park entrance. Park in the Old Trout Farm parking area to the right of the visitor center. **Trailhead Access**

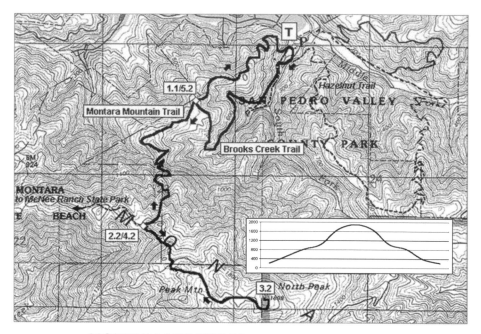

MONTARA MOUNTAIN

Route Directions Follow signs to Brooks Creek and Montara Mountain trails from Old Trout Farm parking area. Veer left on **Brooks Creek Trail**. Stay right on Brooks Creek Trail.

1.1 Turn left on **Montara Mountain Trail**.

2.2 Turn left on **McNee Ranch State Park Montara Mountain Trail**.

3.2 North Peak; turnaround point.

4.2 Turn right on **Montara Mountain Trail**.

5.2 Continue straight on Montara Mountain Trail at junction with Brooks Creek Trail.

About the Trail Begin this semi-loop trip on the Brooks Creek Trail, a singletrack that starts to climb in a large stand of eucalyptus. On a moderate uphill grade, the smooth dirt trail emerges onto open slopes, where coastal scrub—coffeeberry, sticky monkeyflower, evergreen huckleberry, and ceanothus—dominate the vegetation. Manzanita arcs over the trail, forming a tunnel of red-barked, twisted branches, and cow parsnip, forget-me-not, blackberry, and thimbleberry grow in lusher patches of the hillside. The deep ravine of South Fork San Pedro Creek cleaves the slope below you.

You have your first views of the coast—from Pacifica to Marin—where you turn left to join the Montara Mountain Trail. The trail levels temporarily before beginning to climb switchbacks up the steep side of Montara Mountain. Rocks and an uneven trail make footing more difficult as you near McNee Ranch State Park. With one eye on the trail, look west with the other to catch glimpses of the panoramic view.

You cross into McNee Ranch State Park and continue toward the peak on the Montara Mountain Trail, now a wide fire trail. This final stretch before you reach the peak is gradual but exposed, and fog, heat, or wind could make the ascent less enjoyable if you aren't prepared. On clear days, you'll have far-reaching views: Montara Beach and the San Mateo coastline lie southwest, beyond coastal ridges; the blue expanse of the Pacific stretches to the horizon; and Mt. Diablo rises northeast across the bay, beyond the East Bay hills. The trail crosses protruding granite slabs and pebbled sand where the granite has weathered significantly. Manzanita, ceanothus, coyote bush, and ferns flank the trail's sides. Raptors circle the mountain in search of prey. The climb culminates at North Peak with 360-degree views of the Bay Area.

On the return, stretch your legs on this gentle downhill before re-entering San Pedro Valley Park. Watch for the right turn onto the Montara Mountain Trail from McNee Ranch State Park—it's easy to miss. Return to the trailhead all the way on the Montara Mountain Trail. At first steep and rocky, the descent eases and then ends on switchbacks through a eucalyptus forest.

Alternate Routes

If you're not up to the 1700-foot climb to North Peak, other trails in San Pedro Valley Park provide less strenuous routes. The Hazelnut Trail and Weiler Ranch Road Trail compose a loop of about 5 miles. For a slightly longer loop, add the 1.6-mile Valley View Trail.

Trail Notes

• Singletrack and fire trails
• Some rocky sections on singletrack Montara Mountain Trail
• No dogs
• No bikes on this route in San Pedro Valley Park; bikes allowed in McNee Ranch State Park
• No horses

- Bathroom at trailhead; water fountain may not work
- $4 parking fee
- Maps available at visitor center

 Your options are limited, but the shopping center at the corner of Linda Mar Blvd. and Highway 1 in Pacifica is the closest place to find food.

Nature Notes You'll notice exposed granite slabs along the trail as you near Montara Mountain's North Peak. The mountain's granitic rock was formed about 80 million years ago, far south of where it now stands. Montara Mountain, like Point Reyes, rests on the Pacific Plate, which is separated from the North American Plate by the San Andreas fault. The fault runs the length of California; it leaves terra firma at Mussel Rock (just north of Pacifica in Daly City), crosses the Golden Gate under water, and returns to land at Bolinas Lagoon in Marin County. Geologic activity along the fault has forced the Pacific Plate northward for millennia, and continues to do so. The present location and unique rock composition of Montara Mountain testify to California's geologic process.

SAN BRUNO MOUNTAIN STATE AND COUNTY PARK

The low crest of 1314-foot San Bruno Mountain, a familiar land-mark for travelers to and from the San Francisco International Airport, forms the far northern tip of the Santa Cruz Mountains. From a distance San Bruno Mountain appears to be a barren mass, yet this 2326-acre island of open space among the sea of box houses and urban development is home to thriving and diverse plant and animal life. A quick drive from the peninsula, San Francisco, and even the East Bay, the mountain is an unlikely haven where you can enjoy outstanding views of the Bay Area and discover rare plants along its 12 miles of trails.

What You'll Find

San Bruno Mountain State and County Park opens at 8 AM; closing hours vary seasonally—call for details. No dogs are allowed in the park. Bikes and horses are allowed on limited trails. Restrooms and water are available at the park entrance. There is a $4 parking fee.

50

EAST PEAK LOOP
AND RIDGELINE

On rocky singletrack and fire trails, you'll climb to the peak and then run out-and-back along a gently undulating ridge. This route tours San Bruno Mountain's diverse micro-environments and highlights the striking contrast between the mountain's natural world and the adjacent urban and industrial sprawl. Brilliant views on clear days and impressive early-spring wildflower displays are some of the mountain's attractions.

Distance	7.3 miles
Time	1–1.75 hours
Type	semi-loop
High Point/Low Point	1223′/603′
Difficulty	moderate
Use	light
Maps	map at trailhead and entrance kiosk
Area Management	San Mateo County Parks and Recreation Division

Trailhead Access
From Hwy. 101, take the Bayshore Blvd. exit and turn west on Guadalupe Canyon Pkwy. After 1.5 miles, turn right into the park entrance.

From Hwy. 280 southbound, take the Eastmoor Ave. exit and turn left on Sullivan Ave. Make the first left turn onto San Pedro Rd. and cross the freeway. San Pedro Rd. turns into East Market St., which turns into Guadalupe Canyon Pkwy. Turn right into the park entrance.

From Hwy. 280 northbound, take the Mission St. exit. Turn left at the first stop sign onto Junipero Serra Blvd. Turn right on San Pedro Rd. and follow the directions above.

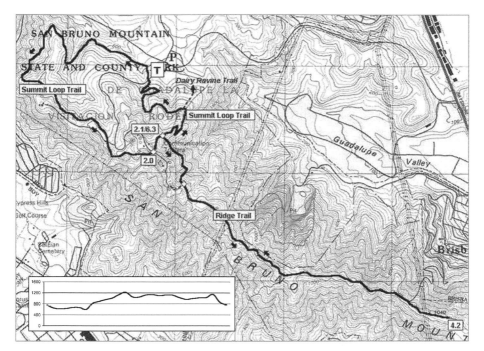

EAST PEAK LOOP AND RIDGELINE

Walk up paved Radio Rd. from parking lot. Cross Guadalupe **Route** Canyon Pkwy. via underpass. Begin on right-branching (northeast) **Directions** **Summit Loop Trail,** just past Native Plant Garden (on left).

1.8 Cross paved road and continue east on Summit Loop Trail.

2.0 Cross paved Radio Rd. at radio towers and continue on Summit Loop Trail on other side.

2.1 Turn right on **Ridge Trail** (beginning out-and-back portion).

2.2 Turn left on Ridge Trail to East Peak at junction with trail to summit vista.

4.2 East Peak turnaround (sign reads 2.0 miles). Retrace route back to junction with Summit Loop Trail.

6.3 Turn right on **Summit Loop Trail.** Pass Dairy Ravine and Eucalyptus Loop trails.

The singletrack Summit Loop Trail traverses the eastern flank of the **About the** mountain on a gradual climb to the summit. As you begin, tall cof- **Trail** feeberry shrubs and cow parsnip hem the trail, and sword ferns, grasses, and gumweed line the lower border. Cars on Guadalupe

Canyon Parkway are loud initially, but their disruption fades as you head up the mountain. Cross April Brook on a wooden bridge and follow the low ravine of the creek eastward up the slope. Arroyo willows, sticky monkeyflower, fragrant California sagebrush, low-lying honeysuckle, and the pale-yellow spring blossoms of wallflowers flank the trail. Rich, earthen smells rise from the creek-dampened soil, and you may see rabbits darting across the trail.

As you approach the summit, the trail becomes rockier, and coyote bush, lupine, and California sagebrush dominate the drier hillside; purple Douglas iris also add spring color. Your views broaden and you take in San Francisco, the East Bay, and the coast (beyond the row houses of Colma).

You cross the paved radio-tower area at the summit and pick up the Ridge Trail on the other side. It begins as a singletrack and soon becomes a wide trail over embedded rock that can make footing unstable. You can see the trail ahead of you, along the mountain's east ridge. The slopes ripple into the city below. Coyote bush and ceanothus pervade the air with their strong fragrance, and purple checkerbloom and bright orange poppies grace the trail in spring. The east peak turnaround point is at 2.4 miles, (although a sign incorrectly indicates 2.0 miles), where the peak slopes steeply to the Hitachi building and a small marina north of the San Francisco Airport.

Retrace your steps along the Ridge Trail and join the Summit Loop Trail, a rocky singletrack. You descend through coyote bush, stands of rushes, and fields of Douglas iris and delicate white milkmaids that coat the hillside as early as February. The trail ends at the native plant garden next to the paved road from the parking area.

Alternate Routes For a shorter run, skip the Summit Loop Trail and park at the top of Radio Road to run the Ridge Trail, 4.8 miles round trip. Or skip the Ridge Trail and traverse the Dairy Ravine, Eucalyptus, and/or Summit Loop trails on the flanks of the mountain.

Trail Notes
- Singletrack and wide trails
- Rocky sections on Ridge Trail
- No dogs
- Bikes only on paved roads on this route
- Horses allowed on all trails, but very uncommon

- Restrooms at parking area, south side of Guadalupe Canyon Parkway
- $4 parking fee

Beyond the scattered stands of sourgrass and the obvious swath of eucalyptus trees that cross the mountain, San Bruno Mountain holds many plant treasures. This richly vegetated sanctuary for native plants is home to some 14 rare and endangered species, including Franciscan wallflower (*Erysimum franciscanum*), San Francisco Owl's Clover (*Orthocarpus floribundus*), and San Bruno Mountain Manzanita (*Arctostaphylos imbricata*). The mountain is also home to four endangered or threatened butterfly species: the San Bruno Elfin, Mission Blue, Callippe Silverspot, and Bay Checkerspot. A Habitat Conservation Plan adopted in the mid-1980s ensures the protection of the endangered species and their habitats. Devoted volunteers maintain a propagation garden for native plants at the base of the mountain.

Nature Notes

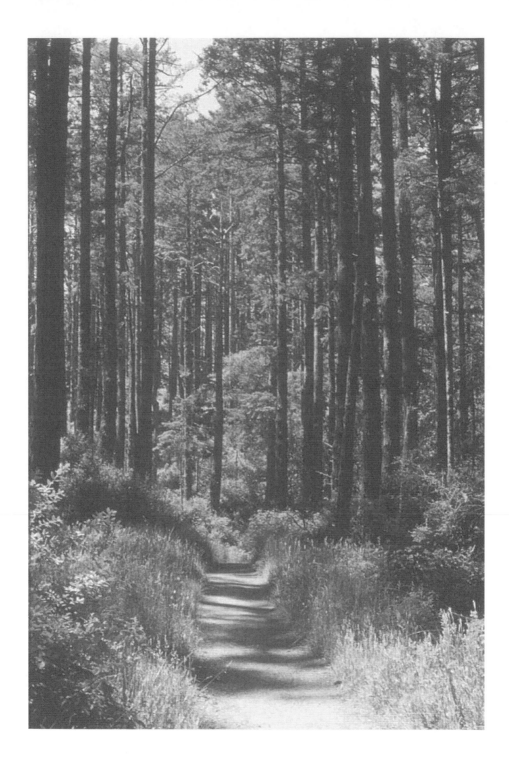

CONTACTS FOR PARKS AND MANAGING AGENCIES

SAN FRANCISCO

Golden Gate National Recreation Area
   visitor center (415) 561-4728
Angel Island State Park
   (415) 435-1915; www.angelisland.org

MARIN

Marin Municipal Water District
   Sky Oaks Ranger Station (415) 945-1181
   Kiosk at entrance to Lake Lagunitas/Bon Tempe
   (415) 945-1182
Mount Tamalpais State Park
   Pantoll Ranger Station (415) 388-2070
Samuel P. Taylor State Park
   (415) 488-9897
Golden Gate National Recreation Area
   Marin Headlands visitor center at Rodeo Beach/
   Fort Cronkhite (415) 331-1540
Point Reyes National Seashore
   Bear Valley visitor center (415) 464-5100
Marin County Open Space District
   (415) 499-6387
Muir Woods
   (415) 388-2595

EAST BAY

East Bay Regional Park District
   EBRPD Headquarters (510) 562-PARK (24-hour
   information); www.ebparks.org

Opposite page:
Sky Trail,
Point Reyes
National Seashore
(Run 17)

City of Oakland, Department of Parks and Recreation
Joaquin Miller Park (510) 482-7857
University of California, Berkeley, Campus Facilities Services
642-6648
East Bay Municipal Utility District
Orinda Watershed Headquarters
500 San Pablo Dam Road
(510) 287-0459 or (925) 254-3778

PENINSULA

Pescadero Creek County Park Complex
Memorial County Park (information for Pescadero)
(650) 879-0238
San Mateo County Parks and Recreation (650) 363-4021
Midpeninsula Regional Open Space District
(650) 691-1200; mrosd@openspace.org
San Bruno Mountain State and County Park
(650) 992-6770
San Pedro County Park
visitor center (650) 355-8289
Wunderlich County Park
(650) 851-1210

MAP CONTACTS

The Olmstead & Bros. Map Co.
Box 5351
Berkeley, CA 94705
(510) 658-6534
Pease Press
1717 Cabrillo Street
San Francisco, CA 94121
(415) 387-1437
benpease@mindspring.com
Tom Harrison Maps
2 Falmouth Cove
San Rafael, CA 94901-4465
(415) 456-7940 or (800) 265-9090
www.tomharrisonmaps.com

RUNS FOR EVERY TYPE OF RUNNER, WEATHER, AND SCENERY

Suggested runs in this book when looking for:

FLAT

Strawberry Canyon Fire Trail, **Run 35**
Joaquin Miller Loop, **Run 36**
Blithedale Ridge, **Run 19**
Kent Lake Out-and-Back, **Run 13**
Windy Hill Ridgeline, **Run 45**

HILL WORKOUTS

Ohlone Wilderness Trail Loop, **Run 30**
Cave Rocks Loop, **Run 31**
Briones Crest Loop, **Run 28**
Upper San Leandro Reservoir and Ridge Loop, **Run 33**
Lafayette Reservoir, **Run 34**

GREAT SINGLETRACK TRAILS

Huckleberry Trail (Blithedale Ridge, **Run 19**)
Yolanda Trail (Phoenix Lake Loop, **Run 10**)
French Trail (Redwood Regional Park, **Run 25**)
Coast Trail (Pantoll Loop, **Run 9**)
Kent Trail (Alpine Lake Traverse, **Run 11**)
Greenpicker Trail (Olema Valley to the Coast, **Run 16**)
Resolution Trail (El Corte de Madera Loop, **Run 48**)
Meadow Trail (Bear Valley Loop, **Run 17**)
Bella Vista Trail (Black Mountain Loop at Monte Bello, **Run 41**)

DOGS (ON- AND OFF-LEASH)

East Bay Regional Park District (except Coyote Hills), **Runs 22–31**
Marin Municipal Water District land, **Runs 10–13**
Coal Creek Preserve, **Run 43**
Ocean Beach, **Run 3**
Strawberry Canyon Fire Trail, **Run 35**
Windy Hill Preserve, **Runs 44 and 45**
Marin County Open Space District, **Runs 19–21**
Bolinas Ridge, **Run 14**

COOL ROUTES FOR HOT DAYS

El Corte de Madera Loop, **Run 48**
Old Haul Road, **Run 37**
French Trail Loop, **Run 25**
Joaquin Miller Loop, **Run 36**

LONG ROUTE POSSIBILITIES

East Bay Skyline National Trail: A 31-mile trail through 6 regional
parks, including Wildcat Canyon, Tilden, Redwood, and
Anthony Chabot. See **Runs 22–27, 30, and 31.**
Ohlone Wilderness Trail: A 28-mile trail from Mission Peak in
Hayward to Del Valle Regional Park. See Ohlone Wilderness
Trail Loop, **Run 30**
Bolinas Ridge: An 11-mile trail from Mt. Tamalpais to Point Reyes
National Seashore. See **Run 14.**

EASY ACCESS FROM URBAN AREAS

Rush Creek, **Run 21**
Rancho San Antonio, **Run 38**
Crissy Field to Baker Beach, **Run 1**
Lands End, **Run 2**
Ocean Beach to Fort Funston, **Run 3**
Angel Island, **Run 4**
Rodeo Valley Loop, **Run 5**
Gerbode Valley Loop, **Run 6**
Green Gulch Loop, **Run 7**
East Peak Loop and Ridgeline, **Run 50**

COAST

Pantoll Loop, **Run 9**
Green Gulch, **Run 7**
Palomarin, **Run 15**
Ocean Beach, **Run 3**
Lands End, **Run 2**
Olema Valley to the Coast, **Run 16**

REDWOODS

West Ridge Loop, **Run 24**
French Trail Loop, **Run 25**
El Corte de Madera Loop, **Run 48**
Mountain Home Loop, **Run 8**

VIEWS

Angel Island, **Run 4**
Pantoll Loop, **Run 9**
Barnabe Mountain, **Run 18**
Meadows Canyon and Big Springs Loop, **Run 23**

SPRING WILDFLOWERS

Russian Ridge, **Run 42**
Mt. Burdell, **Run 20**
Pantoll Loop, **Run 9**
Phoenix Lake Loop, **Run 10**
Ohlone Wilderness Loop, **Run 30**
Cave Rocks Loop, **Run 31**
East Peak Loop and Ridgeline, **Run 50**
Gerbode Valley Loop, **Run 6**

PEACEFUL AND PASTORAL

Bolinas Ridge, **Run 14**
Mt. Burdell, **Run 20**
Briones Crest Loop, **Run 28**

OF GEOLOGIC INTEREST

Northside Loop, **Run 12**
Pantoll Loop, **Run 9** (Benstein Trail)
Alpine Lake Traverse, **Run 11** (Rocky Ridge Fire Road)
Cave Rocks Loop, **Run 31**
El Corte de Madera Loop, **Run 48**
Rodeo Valley, **Run 3**

WETLANDS

Rush Creek, **Run 21**
Coyote Hills Roundabout, **Run 29**

TRAIL RUNNING RESOURCES

Information about running abounds—a trip to the library, the bookstore, or a quick search on the web will unearth endless books, clubs, races, and websites with facts and advice about every aspect of running. The following resources are focused specifically on trail running (with a couple broader websites thrown in).

BOOKS

Boulbol, Scott, Monique Cole and Phil Mislinski. *Trail Runner's Guide to Colorado: 50 Great Trail Runs.* Golden, CO: Fulcrum Publishing, 1999.

Chase, Adam W., and Nancy Hobbs. *The Ultimate Guide to Trail Running: Everything You Need to Know About Equipment, Finding Trails, Nutrition, Hill Strategy, Racing, Training, Weather, First Aid, and Much More.* Guilford, CT: The Lyons Press, 2001.

McQuaide, Mike. *Trail Running Guide to Western Washington.* Seattle, WA: Sasquach Books, 2001.

Shahin, Samir, Stan Swartz, and Jim Wolff. *50 Trail Runs in Southern California.* Seattle, WA: The Mountaineers, 2000.

WEBSITES

All American Trail Running Association www.trailrunner.com
Trail Runner Magazine www.trailrunnermag.com
On the Run www.ontherun.com
The Schedule www.theschedule.com

LOCAL TRAIL RACES

Bay Area UltraRunners races www.home.earthlink.net/~anncarl/
The Dipsea Race www.dipsea.org
Enviro Sports Environmental Outings www.envirosports.com

Lake Chabot Trail Challenge www.trailchallenge.com
Pacific Coast Trail Runs www.pacifictrailruns.com
Redwood Trails www.redwoodtrails.com

BAY AREA RUNNING CLUBS

Dolphin South End Runners www.dserunners.com
East Bay Striders www.eastbaystriders.org
Hoys Excelsior Running Club
    http://tkecapital.com/hoys-excelsior.htm
Golden Bay Runners www.goldenbayrunners.org
Mission Peak Striders www.mpstriders.com
Palo Alto Run Club www.parunclub.com
Tamalpa Runners www.tamalparunners.org

EQUIPMENT

Athleta Women's Sports Apparel www.athleta.com
Road Runner Sports www.roadrunnersports.com
Title 9 Sports www.title9sports.com

BAY AREA RUNNING STORES

Fleet Feet, San Francisco and Capitola
Hoys, San Francisco
On the Run, San Fransisco
The Runners High, Menlo Park and Los Altos
Transport, Oakland

SELECTED SOURCES AND RECOMMENDED READING

NATURAL HISTORY

Alt, David D., and Hyndman, Donald W. *Roadside Geology of Northern California*. Missoula, MT: Mountain Press Publishing Co., 1975.

Bakker, Elna. *An Island Called California*. 2nd ed. Berkeley, CA: University of California Press, 1984.

Castle Rock State Park. [pamphlet] California State Parks, and Portola and Castle Rock Foundation, 2000.

Evens, Jules C. *The Natural History of the Point Reyes Peninsula*. Point Reyes, CA: Point Reyes National Seashore Association, 1988.

Gilliam, Harold. Weather of the San Francisco Bay Region. 2nd ed. Berkeley, CA: University of California Press, 2002.

Hill, Mary. *California Landscape: Origin and Evolution*. Berkeley, CA: University of California Press, 1984.

Howard, Arthur David. *Evolution of the Landscape of the San Francisco Bay Region*. Berkeley, CA: University of California Press, 1962.

Johnson, Sharon G., Pamela C. Muick, Bruce M. Pavlik, and Marjorie Popper. *Oaks of California*. Los Olivos, CA: Cachuma Press, 1991.

Keator, Glenn. *Complete Garden Guide to the Native Shrubs of California*. San Francisco, CA: Chronicle Books, 1994.

Smith, Arthur C. *Introduction to the Natural History of the San Francisco Bay Region*. Berkeley, CA: University of California Press, 1959.

GUIDEBOOKS

Heid, Matt. *101 Hikes in Northern California*. Berkeley, CA: Wilderness Press, 2000.

Liberatore, Karen. *The Complete Guide to the Golden Gate National Recreation Area*. San Francisco, CA: Chronicle Books, 1982.

Margolin, Malcolm. *The East Bay Out*. Revised ed. Berkeley, CA: Heyday Books, 1988.

Martin, Don and Kay. *Hiking Marin: 121 Great Hikes in Marin County*. San Anselmo, CA: Martin Press, 1995.

———*Mt. Tam: A Hiking, Running, and Nature Guide*. San Anselmo, CA: Martin Press, 1986.

——— *Point Reyes National Seashore: A Hiking and Nature Guide*. San Anselmo, CA: Martin Press, 1992.

Ornduff, Robert. *Introduction to California Plant Life*. Berkeley, CA: University of California Press, 1974.

Rusmore, Jean. *Peninsula Trails: Outdoor Adventures on the San Francisco Peninsula*. 3rd ed. Berkeley, CA: Wilderness Press, 1997.

———*The Bay Area Ridge Trail: Ridgetop Adventures Above San Francisco Bay*. Berkeley, CA: Wilderness Press, 1995.

Rusmore, Jean, Betsy Crowder and Frances Spangle. *South Bay Trails: Outdoor Adventures in & around Santa Clara County*. 3rd ed. Berkeley, CA: Wilderness Press, 2001.

Spitz, Barry. *Tamalpais Trails*. San Anselmo, CA: Potrero Meadow Publishing Company, 1990.

Taber, Tom. *The Santa Cruz Mountains Trail Book*. 7th ed. San Mateo, CA: The Oak Valley Press, 1994.

Wayburn, Peggy. *Adventuring in the San Francisco Bay Area: The Sierra Club Travel Guide to San Francisco, Marin, Sonoma, Napa, Solano, Contra Costa, Alameda, Santa Clara, San Mateo Counties, and the Bay Islands*. San Francisco, CA: Sierra Club Books, 1987.

Weintraub, David. *East Bay Trails: Outdoor Adventures in Alameda and Contra Costa Counties*. Berkeley, CA: Wilderness Press, 1998.

———*North Bay Trails: Outdoor Adventures in Marin, Napa, & Sonoma counties*. Berkeley, CA: Wilderness Press, 1999.

Whitnah, Dorothy. *Point Reyes: A Guide to the Trails, Roads, Beaches, Campgrounds, and Lakes of Point Reyes National Seashore*. 3rd ed. Berkeley, CA: Wilderness Press, 1997.

———*Guide to the Golden Gate National Recreation Area*. Berkeley, CA: Wilderness Press, 1978.

MAPS

Hiking, Bicycling, and Equestrian Trail Map of the Central Peninsula. Palo Alto, CA: The Trail Center.

Hiking, Bicycling, and Equestrian Trail Map of the Southern Peninsula. Palo Alto, CA: The Trail Center, 1996.

Trails of the East Bay Hills: Central Section, including Redwood, Chabot,

Las Trampas, Sibley, and Joaquin Miller Parks and Lands of East Bay M.U.D. Berkeley, CA: The Olmstead & Bros. Map Co.

Trails of the East Bay Hills: Northern Section, including Tilden, Wildcat Canyon and Briones Parks and Lands of East Bay M.U.D. Berkeley, CA: The Olmstead & Bros. Map Co.

Trails of Mt. Tamalpais and the Marin Headlands: Complete Guide to Hiking, Biking, and Horse Trails. Berkeley, CA: The Olmstead & Bros. Map Co.

Trails of Northeast Marin County. San Francisco, CA: Pease Press.

Peninsula Parklands: Where to Hike, Bicycle, Ride, Picnic, and Camp in San Francisco, San Mateo, Santa Clara, and Santa Cruz Counties, California. 3rd ed. Palo Alto, CA: The Trail Center, 2000.

Point Reyes National Seashore Trail Map. San Rafael, CA: Tom Harrison Maps.

INDEX

ABOUT THE AUTHOR

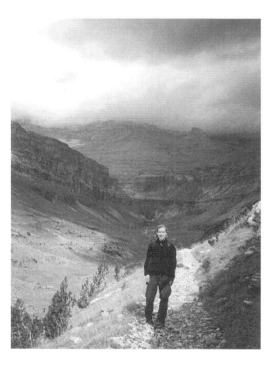

For her debut book, Jessica Lage turns to a subject dear to her heart. *Trail Runner's Guide San Francisco Bay Area* grows out of her passion for nature and the landscapes of her native Bay Area, as well as her long-time devotion to trail running. Fortunate to live a few steps from some of the Bay Area's best trails, Jessica is an avid outdoor enthusiast whose communication skills make her a premier spokesperson for this increasingly popular sport.

Jessica earned a B.A. in American Studies from the University of California, Berkeley, and is currently working on a Master's Degree at the University of Colorado, Boulder, in Geography. Her second book, a guidebook about Point Reyes National Seashore in California, is forthcoming from Wilderness Press.